INFORMATION
MEDICINE

"There are moments in the history of science that profoundly redirect the practice of medicine. It may be that the research findings encountered in this book will rank as an equally memorable moment. If, as seems likely, this research significantly relieves human suffering worldwide, Pier Mario Biava will come to stand in medicine's pantheon alongside giants such as Anton van Leeuwenhoek, William Harvey, Ignaz Semmelweis, and many other visionaries whose insights have diminished human misery and increased the probability that the human spirit will soar."

LARRY DOSSEY, M.D.,
AUTHOR OF *REINVENTING MEDICINE: BEYOND
MIND-BODY TO A NEW ERA OF HEALING*

"This book gifts us in extraordinary ways. It informs us and re-connects us to that pristine in-forming field of reality that underlies our existence. Furthermore, it opens up a field of medical research that has the potential to reorder the entire biological domain, to counteract disease predispositions, reverse disease conditions, and invigorate health."

RAOUL GOLDBERG, M.D., MEDICAL DIRECTOR OF THE
PATH TO HEALTH CANCER CENTER AND AUTHOR OF
*ADDICTIVE BEHAVIOUR IN CHILDREN AND
YOUNG ADULTS* AND *AWAKENING TO CHILD HEALTH*

"*Information Medicine* not only covers the breadth of a new paradigm of regenerative medicine but also reinforces and documents the cutting edge of science that is unfolding before our eyes. It also looks at the science-backed research of how health problems will be treated in the not too distant future. This book is extremely well researched and documented, exhibiting a range and breadth of knowledge ranging from vibrational medicine to quantum physics to epigenetics and pluripotent stem cells to reprogram cancer cells. An important contribution to the field of regenerative medicine, a must-read for anyone interested in this topic."

ELISA LOTTOR, PH.D., H.M.D.,
EXPERT IN NUTRITION, HOMEOPATHY, AND ENERGY MEDICINE;
INTERNATIONAL LECTURER; AND
AUTHOR OF *THE MIRACLE OF REGENERATIVE MEDICINE*
AND *FEMALE AND FORGETFUL*

INFORMATION
MEDICINE

THE **REVOLUTIONARY** **CELL-REPROGRAMMING DISCOVERY** THAT **REVERSES CANCER** AND **DEGENERATIVE DISEASES**

ERVIN LASZLO AND PIER MARIO BIAVA, M.D.

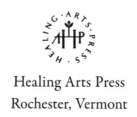

Healing Arts Press
Rochester, Vermont

Healing Arts Press
One Park Street
Rochester, Vermont 05767
www.HealingArtsPress.com

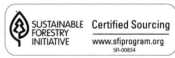

Text stock is SFI certified

Healing Arts Press is a division of Inner Traditions International

*Note to the reader: This book is intended as an informational guide. The remedies,
approaches, and techniques described herein are meant to supplement, and not to be a
substitute for, professional medical care or treatment. They should not be used to treat
a serious ailment without prior consultation with a qualified health care professional.*

Cataloging-in-Publication Data for this title is available from the Library of Congress

ISBN 978-1-62055-822-5 (print)
ISBN 978-1-62055-823-2 (ebook)

Printed and bound in the United States by Lake Book Manufacturing, Inc.
The text stock is SFI certified. The Sustainable Forestry Initiative® program
promotes sustainable forest management.

10 9 8 7 6 5 4 3 2 1

Text design and layout by Virginia Scott Bowman
This book was typeset in Garamond Premier Pro and Avenire with Hypatia Sans
and Trenda used as display typefaces

To send correspondence to the authors of this book, mail a first-class letter to the
authors c/o Inner Traditions • Bear & Company, One Park Street, Rochester, VT
05767, and we will forward the communication, or contact Ervin Laszlo at
http://ervinlaszlo.com and Pier Mario Biava directly at **https://www.biava.me/en**.

Contents

◎

PART ONE
The Breakthrough

CHAPTER III

SUMMING UP: THE MEANING OF INFORMATION MEDICINE FOR OUR LIFE AND TIMES

◎

PART TWO

The Research

Foreword

Deepak Chopra, M.D.

It's a natural part of any discovery to find yourself lying awake at night, settling down from the excitement of a breakthrough, and saying to yourself, "If I'm right, this changes everything." Most of the time, however, everything doesn't change. If the discovery winds up being accepted, you might be fortunate, and a few things will change.

The ideas forwarded in this new book by Ervin Laszlo and Pier Mario Biava are rare, even in a rapidly changing landscape where science is reevaluating time-honored concepts on every side. The seed idea of "in-formation" has the potential to change everything—for real. The first headline that is likely to emerge from the breakthrough described in these pages will focus on cancer. The clinical results with advanced liver-cancer patients detailed in part two are startling. But I'd like to dwell for a moment on the larger implications of "in-formation," because in fact cancer treatments and all the other medical applications described in this book, hugely promising as they are, only hint at a paradigm shift that could break open our accepted notion about what is real.

The "real" reality isn't an issue for 99 percent of working scientists, or a large percentage of nonscientists, because they have found a work-around that keeps daily life flowing in well-worn grooves. Scientists and nonscientists alike navigate the day trusting the evidence of the five senses—accepting as a given the physical world "out there." This is a work-around because the quantum revolution more than a century ago caused the substantial, hard-edged, solid physical world to vanish. What the five senses report, and the notion of tiny, tiny things (atoms and molecules) that pile up to form big, big things (stars and galaxies) was negated once and for all.

This discovery, which has been described endlessly since the pioneering era of Einstein, Heisenberg, Schrödinger, and their brilliant colleagues, got sidelined by everyday life. The entire universe may vanish into an invisible dimension devoid of time, space, matter, and energy, but that obviously isn't visible when you drive your car to work or watch a sunrise. The continuity of the world that we occupy every day undermines any abstruse theory about reality. This has remained true decades after the eminent astronomer and physicist Sir Arthur Eddington drily noted, "It is difficult for the matter-of-fact physicist to accept the view that the substratum of everything is of mental character." And working science, including medicine, has turned its back on the insight of another eminent physicist, Sir James Jeans, who is worth quoting at length: "The universe begins to look more like a great thought than like a great machine. Mind no longer appears to be an accidental intruder into the realm of matter . . . we ought rather to hail it as the creator and governor of the realm of matter."

Laszlo and Biava return us directly to this insight, and the reason their book has a chance to change everything is that they provide an entry into everyday life. They have clinical proof for turning on its head the accepted default that we are biological machines that somehow learned to think. Rather, we are minds that learned how to create a body.

The authors invoke the late British physicist David Bohm, who spent his career maintaining that the visible order observable in the created universe, from the level of quantum activity to the most evolved forms, including human DNA, was controlled by an invisible organizing principle or force. This invisible agency exists outside time and space, but it informs every structure in creation, and to that end Bohm devised the term "in-formation." As intriguing as his idea was—this entire book is devoted to showing exactly how right he happened to be—there was widespread resistance among fellow physicists.

The reasons for this, aside from sheer prejudice and mental laziness, came down to a clash with long-accepted assumptions that formed a kind of Chinese wall against Bohm's insight. One assumption is that matter is more real than mind; another is that reality must be broken down into measurable units. Bohm couldn't actually point to a measurable force or offer any material evidence for in-formation. His chief ally, intellectually speaking, was negative logic. Without in-formation, there was no viable way to explain the intricacies of evolving forms in the universe and the astonishing complexity of their design. But luck wasn't with him in a context where "design" had become a poisoned word in science, thanks to reactionary religious fundamentalists.

Whole books have been devoted to the relationship of mind and matter, how consciousness came about, and where the universe, along with life on Earth, is evolving. Biava and Laszlo have made a wise decision by talking to other scientists, including the medical community, in terms they already accept. Climbing down from the ladder of philosophy, they present hard evidence. Surely this is the right path, for the time being. The Chinese wall that kept Bohm isolated until his death in 1992 won't crumble until consciousness is taken seriously as a viable subject of research, because the terms Bohm had to use in order to communicate—mind, matter, force, agency, and so on—are red herrings when the "real" reality is consciousness.

This book isn't the first to found its ideas on the age-old realization that the two worlds, "in here" and "out there," are entirely created from and by consciousness endlessly changing and yet always maintaining a level of continuity. No matter how different a star, a sea snail, a tree fern, and a newborn baby appear, each is a modification of innate qualities that inhere to consciousness: intelligence, self-awareness, creativity, evolution, and wholeness. All are implied by the term "in-formation," because it is the medium by which every quality of consciousness is made manifest.

In-formation is the invisible glue that keeps your body from flying apart into a whirling cloud of disorganized, chaotic particles, blowing in the wind like a dust storm. In a way, the existence of in-formation is self-evident, making it baffling to look around and see broken-down materialism, outmoded a century ago, still persisting as the default attitude of all but a few. Laszlo and Biava have made a major contribution to the paradigm shift that will inevitably come, and when it arrives, they will deserve a large measure of acknowledgement from all sides.

DEEPAK CHOPRA, M.D., is a world-renowned authority in the field of mind-body healing, a best-selling author, and the founder of the Chopra Center in California. His nonprofit organization, the Chopra Foundation, is dedicated to improving health and well-being, cultivating spiritual knowledge, expanding consciousness, and promoting world peace. Before establishing the Chopra Center and the Chopra Foundation, he served as chief of staff at Boston Regional Medical Center. He received his medical degree from the All India Institute of Medical Sciences and is board certified in internal medicine, endocrinology, and metabolism. He is a fellow of the American College of Physicians and a member of the American Association of Clinical Endocrinologists.

In addition to being well known through his social media presence, Dr. Chopra is the prolific author of more than eighty-five books, including fourteen best sellers, on mind-body health, quantum mechanics, spirituality, and peace. His recent book *The Healing Self* was cowritten with Rudolph E. Tanzi and published in 2018. Dr. Chopra's books have been published in more than forty-three languages.

Preface

The book in the hands of the reader introduces a major discovery in the field of medicine. This discovery is not a unique and disconnected element in the history of medicine: it is a logical corollary of the advance of knowledge in the field of science as a whole. This advance is what we call "the new paradigm." The discovery on which we report here is both a fruit of this advance and a brilliant testimony to its validity. The new discovery in medicine, and therewith science's new paradigm, impacts all aspects of our life. Hence this book is addressed to both the medical professional and to all people concerned with the way we care for our health and treat disease.

Part one introduces the new discovery in medicine as a particular, and particularly important, application of the new paradigm in science. The new paradigm presented in chapter I revisits and revalidates some perennial insights. The living organism is a seamless whole: it is a "cognitive network" that functions by receiving and elaborating information. The information it receives is more than the ensemble of humanly produced messages: it is the cosmic "in-formation" discussed by quantum physicist David Bohm.

The reception and elaboration of "in-formation" in a living system is the key to its health and viability, but this in-formation is not always fully and correctly received. This flaw can be rectified. Chapter II offers a concise review of the groundbreaking experiments, identifying the power of in-formation medicine to treat and cure some hitherto untreatable and incurable diseases. Chapter III offers assessments by leading experts in the field, highlighting the epochal significance of the advent of in-formation medicine.

Part two is dedicated to the documentation and validation of this revolution in medicine, providing the basis for further research and development. It presents the research that has led to the new discovery and discloses the method and the tools for making it an effective instrument for curing disease and maintaining health.

The new discovery could open a new era of well-being for humanity—an era that could free millions from the curse of diseases that make life nasty, brutish, and short, to cite the words of philosopher Thomas Hobbes.

This book has a two-fold message—a basic worldview message of insight into a new (or perhaps merely newly rediscovered) way of perceiving life, health, and disease, and a practical message disclosing the ways we can henceforth maintain health and treat disease. We trust that it will make a meaningful contribution toward achieving better health and a higher quality of life for people wherever they live on this planet.

PART ONE

THE BREAKTHROUGH

CHAPTER I

The New Paradigm in Science and Medicine

We seek the simplest possible scheme of thought that can tie together the observed facts.

ALBERT EINSTEIN

There is a widely discussed "paradigm shift" underway today. It brings a two-fold revolution—actually parallel strands of a radical "evolution." First and most basically, an evolution in our understanding of the fundamental nature of the world. Second, a logically entailed but still largely independently researched evolution in our understanding of the nature of health and disease. We consider both (r)evolutions, and begin with a review of science's emerging understanding of the world.*

The new concept surfacing at the cutting edge of science is radically new and at the same time millennia old. It is new in relation to the dominant paradigm in science and society, but it is old in its "re-cognition" of intuitions that have hallmarked inquiry into the nature of reality for thousands of years.

The classical paradigm is the inheritance of Newtonian physics. In

---

*A more detailed account is given *inter alia* in Ervin Laszlo, *The Self-Actualizing Cosmos* (Rochester, Vt.: Inner Traditions, 2014) and in *What Is Reality? The New Map of Cosmos and Consciousness* (New York: Select Books, 2016).

light of that paradigm the world consists of individual bits of matter interacting in passive space and indifferently flowing time. This view has been challenged by the "relativity revolution" in the first decade of the twentieth century and by the "quantum revolution" in the third. The paradigm emerging today consolidates these revolutions. It sees the world as a whole system in which all things in their ensemble constitute an entangled macroscopic quantum system. The "global realism" of the new paradigm contrasts with the "local realism" of the old. In the old paradigm, all things occupy unique positions in space and time and are affected only by local forces transmitted through mechanistic interactions. By contrast, in the perspective of global realism, all things are instantly and mutually "entangled" across all points of space and intervals of time.

THE NEW PARADIGM IN PHYSICS

In light of the concept emerging at the frontiers of the physical sciences, the universe is not an arena for structures and entities of matter moving in passive space and indifferently flowing time. As astrophysicist James Jeans noted over a hundred years ago, the universe is more like a great thought than like a great rock.

The concept of a thought-like universe is familiar from the annals of history. Philosophers, scientists, and intuitive people in all walks of life have often questioned that the world would be just as it is presented to our senses. The intuition that it is more thought-like than rock- or machine-like proved to be well founded. The universe is not an ensemble of separate bits of matter obeying mechanistic laws, but an intrinsically whole macroscopic quantum system where all things are in-formed and interconnected beyond the conventional bounds of space and time.

In the new paradigm of physics, the things that exist and persist in the world are sets and clusters of vibrating energy. These clusters are what we experience as the physical furnishings of space and time.

The idea of the world as vibration has been known to the classical wisdom traditions. It was present in the Sanskrit concept of Akasha and was taken up in the Vedic texts of India as early as 5000 BCE. In the Vedas its function was identified with *shabda*, the first vibration, the first ripple that constitutes the universe, and also with *spanda*, the "vibration/movement of consciousness." The contemporary Indian scholar I. K. Taimni wrote, "There is a mysterious integrated state of vibration from which all possible kinds of vibrations can be derived by a process of differentiation. That is called *N.da* in Sanskrit. It is a vibration in a medium which may be translated as 'space' in English. But it is not mere empty space but space which, though apparently empty, contains within itself an infinite amount of potential energy."[1]

This traditional notion is sustained and elaborated at the cutting edge of quantum physics. Research on the ultrasmall dimensions of the universe reveals that space is not empty and smooth, but filled with waves and vibration. At the subquantum level physicists do not find anything they could identify as matter. What they find are standing and propagating waves—clusters of stationary and propagating vibration.

Previously scientists assumed that it is matter that vibrates. There is a ground substance that vibrates, and that substance consists of matter-particles and assemblies of matter-particles. The world is material, and vibration is the way matter behaves. But the contrary turned out to be the case. There is no ground substance. The universe is a system of variously complex and coherent clusters of vibrant energy, and matter is just the way the vibrations appear on observation.

The great physicist Max Planck said this clearly. In one of his last lectures in Florence, he noted, "As a man who has devoted his whole life to the most clear-headed science, to the study of matter, I can tell you as a result of my research about atoms this much: There is no matter as such. All matter originates and exists only by virtue of a force which brings the particles of an atom to vibration and holds this most minute solar system of the atom together."[2]

Planck was not alone in stating the concept of the universe as force and vibration. Two years prior to Planck's pronouncement, the maverick genius Nikola Tesla said that if you want to know the secrets of the universe, think in terms of energy, frequency, and vibration.

In the second decade of the twenty-first century, the materialist concept of the physical world has been definitively transcended. The new physics tells us that it is not from bits of matter but from clusters of ordered energy-vibration that the things we find in the world are built. Ordered vibrations make the furnishing of the universe into what it is: a system of coherent entities and processes, rather than a welter of random unconnected events.

The vibrations that surface in the universe are a consequence of the excitation of the ground state of a wider reality. The universe is no longer considered to be all that is. It is the phase and domain of a wider reality we can best call *cosmos*. The excitation of the cosmos was most likely the effect of the Big Bang. The energies released in that singularity polarized the cosmic ground state and brought it into vibration. The phenomena we observe in the space-time universe are clusters of vibrations of the polarized cosmic ground state. The vibrations are spatially as well as temporally related, and their relations introduced space and time into the undifferentiated oneness of the cosmic ground state. The universe we observe is a spatial and temporal domain of spatially and temporally related clusters of vibration.

The vibrations that emerged fill the space-time of the universe. As far as we know, there is no empty space and no empty interval in the universe. Space is a foaming, turbulent medium filled with fields and forces. The term "vacuum" does not apply to it: it is a *plenum*.

The observed, and in principle observable, dimension of the universe is the ensemble of the vibrations resulting from the excitation of the cosmic ground state. Everything we perceive and observe is a pattern or cluster of vibration created by the excitation of that primordial state. The known and knowable clusters range in size and complexity from quarks and quanta to biological organisms, and from biospheres and planets to galaxies and the metagalaxy. They are particulate entities, but their particularity does not signify separateness. The clusters of vibration in and of the ground state are nonlocal. They are locally differentiated but globally "entangled" elements of the sea of vibration that patterns the ground state of the cosmos.

THE NEW PARADIGM OF EVOLUTION

An estimated 13.8 billion years before our time, the Big Bang excited the ground state of the cosmos and produced ripples in what must have been a seamless primordial state. The ripples were sets of vibrations of coinciding phase and frequency, forming cognizable and re-cognizable "things" against a "background" of undifferentiated, seemingly chaotic vibration. The thinglike clusters interacted and created ever larger and more structured and differentiated "macro-things." These are what we perceive as the material furnishings of the universe. They come into being in the processes of progressive ordering and structuring we call evolution.

Evolution took off in the universe following the inflow of the staggering energies released by the Big Bang. Coherent clusters of vibrations were created, and they produced integral, relatively enduring clusters. Physicists know these clusters as *leptons* (electrons, muons, tau particles, and neutrinos), *mesons* (pions), and *hadrons* (baryons, including protons and neutrons). In the course of time they formed more complex clusters: the atoms of the elements. Atoms in turn clustered into molecules and molecular assemblies. The clusters that appeared as quantized microparticles attracted or repulsed one another and created larger and more complex entities. On the astronomical level these appear to us as stars, stellar systems, and galaxies.

Evolution manifests in perceptible form the ensemble of the laws and regularities that make the universe into what it is: a nonrandom, and at least partly intelligible, domain of space and time.

In modern science, thanks to the work of Darwin and Wallace, evolution was first recognized in the domains of life. Its recognition as a cosmological process had to wait until the first decades of the twentieth century, when Einstein's hopes for an eternally unchanging matrix-universe proved illusory and time entered as a factor in the cosmological equations. Through the work of physicists such as Willem De Sitter and Stephen Hawking, and of thermodynamicists Ilya Prigogine and Aharon Katchalsky, nonlinear but overall irreversible change came to be seen as fundamental in the universe. It appeared that evolution encompasses not just the living world, but the world as a whole.

The factor in the cosmos that structured and evolved first the physical and then the living world was not clearly understood. Physicist Henri Bergson speculated that it is an *élan vital* that counters the trend toward energy-degradation in complex systems, and biologist Hans Driesch suggested that it is a counter-entropic drive he termed *entelechy*. Philosophers Teilhard de Chardin and Erich Jantsch postulated a dynamic tendency called *syntony*, and others spoke of the structuring factor as *syntropy*. Eastern thinkers identified it with the Sanskrit term *prana,* a cosmic energy that permeates all things, and in the West psychoanalyst Wilhelm Reich's concept of *orgone* proved to be a close approximation, the same as spiritual philosopher Rudolf Steiner's *etheric force.* Newton himself recognized the presence of this factor and sought to integrate it with his mechanistic laws. The mechanical laws, he said, are not full descriptions of reality; they need to be completed with the recognition of an "enlivening and ensouling spirit in all things"—a spirit of "vegetation" in the Latin sense of "animating" and "enlivening."[3]

The nature of this universal structuring factor has not been definitively established; current definitions remain controversial. However, that such a factor is present in the universe appears to be beyond reasonable doubt. In the most general and least speculative definition we can call it an "attractor" acting on systems in space and time.

The presence of such an attractor is supported by observation. The systems we observe in the universe cannot have been the result of a random concatenation of disconnected elements. There must have been "something" that biased random interactions and created a trend toward structure, form, and coherence. The observed universe is highly, indeed staggeringly, coherent. This is not likely to be the product of random interactions, no matter how widespread and enduring they may be. A dynamic attractor appears to be at work, biasing the interplay of otherwise random interactions.

This concept comes from physics, where an attractor is defined in reference to the state or behavior toward which a dynamic system tends in space and time. Consider a dynamic system such as a living organism, an ecology, or even an economy. That system is changing over time. If the change does not follow a discernible logic, the system is chaotic and not representable by attractors. But if a logic can be discovered in the evolution of the "phase-space" of the system—its sequence of states or behaviors—then that system can be represented by one or more attractors. The attractors define the state or condition toward which the sequence of states or behaviors tends. If the sequence exhibits elements of repetition over time, the attractor is said to be "periodic." If it exhibits a tendency toward a single state or behavior, the system can be represented by a "point attractor." The evolution of the system can be complex, including unpredictable elements and incomprehensible sequences. In that case, the attractor is said to be "strange" or "chaotic." A complex system can obey diverse attractors at the same time.

Rather than speaking of a higher will or purpose, or of an unexplained élan vital, prana, or etheric force, we can least speculatively assert that the nonrandom evolution of systems in the universe—and the evolution of the macrostructures of the universe themselves—is governed by attractors.

The presence of an attractor that biases interactions in the universe toward complexity and coherence is clearly evident. The universe we observe cannot be the product of mere chance. Already in the middle of the twentieth century physicists Arthur Eddington and Paul Dirac noted curious "coincidences" among the basic physical constants of the universe. For example, the ratio of the electric force to the gravitational force, which is approximately 10^{40}, is matched by the ratio between the size of the universe and the dimension of elementary particles: that ratio, too, is approximately 10^{40}. It is not evident how these ratios could have been produced, and then maintained, by random processes. The ratio of the electric force to the gravitational force should be unchanging (as these forces are constant), whereas the ratio of the size of the universe to the size of elementary particles should be changing (since the universe is expanding). In his "large number hypothesis," Dirac speculated that the agreement between these ratios, one variable and the other not, is more than coincidence. Either the universe is not expanding or the force of gravitation varies with its expansion.

Cosmological research unearthed an entire array of similarly mind-boggling elements of coherence. The mass of elementary particles, the number of particles, and the forces between them display harmonic ratios. Many of the ratios among basic parameters can be interpreted on the one hand in reference to the relationship between the mass of elementary particles and the number of nucleons (particles of the atomic nucleus) in the universe, and on the other in reference to the relationship between the gravitational constant (the factor of gravitation in the evolution of the universe), the charge of the electron, Planck's constant (a unit of measurement used to calculate the smallest measurable time interval and physical distance), and the speed of light.

Also the microwave background radiation—the remnant of the Big Bang—turned out to be unexpectedly coherent. When one maps its sequence of values, there are peaks and troughs, and these follow a definite, nonrandom logic. There is a large peak followed by smaller, harmonic peaks. The series of peaks ends at the longest wavelength that physicist Lee Smolin termed R. When R is divided by the speed of light we get the length of time that independent estimates tell us is the age of the universe. When we divide the speed of light by the value of R (c/R), we get the frequency that equates to one cycle over the age of the universe. And when R is squared and divided by the speed of light (R^2/c), we get the value equal to the acceleration of the expansion of the distant galaxies.

These observations are more than coincidental. The universe is coherent beyond expectation, and its coherence allows life to emerge on suitable surfaces. Life requires a universe of which the basic parameters—the "physical constants"—are precisely and enduringly correlated. Variation of the order of one-billionth of the value of some of these constants (such as the mass of elementary particles, the speed of light, the rate of expansion of galaxies, and two dozen others) would have resulted in a sterile, lifeless universe. Even a minute variation would have prevented the creation of stable atoms and stable relations among them, and this would have precluded the evolution of the complex systems that manifest the characteristics of life. Yet living systems show up in more and more places in the universe, under more and more diverse conditions.

The clusters of vibration that are the fundamental reality of the universe create in-phase, harmoniously structured ensembles that observers such as the human perceive as material—more exactly, matter-like—structures. It appears that the universe evolves under the influence of coherence-generating dynamic attractors. What we observe today is a highly coherent ensemble of clusters of vibration, appearing to us as a universe of staggeringly coherent quasi-material structures.

Not only is the universe as a whole a system of coherent structures; it is also the ground or template for the evolution of a vast array of subsidiary ensembles of coherent clusters of vibration—coherent structures, ranging in size and complexity from atoms to galaxies. These complex and yet coherent clusters could not have come about through a random mixing of their components. Statistical analysis of the complexity of even relatively simple biological systems indicates that to produce them by a random mixing of their components would have taken on the average longer than the age of the universe.

The complexity of the DNA-mRNA-tRNA-rRNA transcription and translation system is such that the probability that living systems would have been produced by random processes is astronomically improbable. Its probability, according to mathematical physicist Fred Hoyle, is equal to that of a hurricane blowing through a scrapyard and assembling a working airplane. Even 13.8 billion years for the evolution of matter-like structures in the physical domain and four billion or more years for the appearance of living systems are not sufficient to account for the presence of stars and galaxies, and the complex and supremely harmonious web of life on this planet.

If random interactions cannot account for the existence of the coherent complex systems we encounter in the universe, we need to recognize the presence of attractors acting on phenomena in space and time. The explanation of their origins and nature is secondary to the affirmation that they exist. Their existence is consistent with the quantum theory developed by physicist David Bohm. According to Bohm, the observed "explicate order" is "in-formed" by the underlying "implicate order." The implicate order is the attractor that governs—"in-forms" in Bohm's theory—the unfolding of events in the explicate order.

The implicate order is the beyond-space-time domain of laws and regularities that govern events in space and time. These laws and regularities are "beyond" the space-time universe in the sense in which the laws of chess, for example, are beyond the games played according to those laws. The laws govern the way the games are played but are not part of the games. They do not physically move the pieces on the board—rather, they regulate the way the pieces can be legitimately moved. The effect of the implicate order on the explicate order is in the form of "active information"—meaning "in-formation." It does not involve physical action such as the action of a force field, whether electric, magnetic, gravitational, or nuclear.

The effect of the attractors (that is, of the implicate order) is universal: it in-forms the entire space-time domain. It is irreducible and illimitable: there are no entities or processes that could be shielded and exempted from it. It is the governing, ordering, and structuring factor religious-spiritual traditions identify as the will of God, Tao, Brahman, or the Great Spirit. It is the factor that makes the universe what it is: an evolving nonrandom system of individually as well as collectively coherent entities and events. In the here suggested conceptual frame, it is the formative ("in-forming") action of dynamic attractors on the space-time universe.

INFORMATION MEDICINE: THE NEW PARADIGM IN HEALTH AND HEALING

Things and events in the universe are not haphazard and chaotic: they are formed—"in-formed"—by universal attractors. The recognition that the manifest world, and thus the living organism, is "in-formed," suggests a new definition of bodily health and disease.

The New Definition of Health and Disease

Health is the full (or at any rate adequate) condition of in-formation in the living organism. Disease is the condition of blocked, reduced, or otherwise flawed in-formation. Healing, then, is the reestablishment of the condition of full (or adequate) in-formation.

The task of medicine is to heal by reestablishing a condition of adequate in-formation in the organism. This does not necessarily call for artificial measures; in many cases, it can be performed by recourse to the in-formation already present in nature. In the global context, doing so is to access and abide by what the religions call the will of a supreme intelligence. In the context of healing, it is equivalent to accessing what the Eastern healing arts name the *chi* or *qi* of the organism.

The living organism is an irreducibly whole system, with all its parts and elements nonlocally—intrinsically and instantly—interconnected. A blockage or other flaw in any part of the organism is not confined to that part. Whatever happens in a cell or in an organ of the organism also happens in all its cells and organs. A cellular or organic malfunction in one part indicates a flaw in the functioning of the organism as a whole.

A healthy organism is intrinsically as well as extrinsically coherent. Its intrinsic coherence comes to light in the cooperation of all its cells, organs, and organ systems in maintaining the whole organism in the living state. Conflict or disharmony between the organism and any part of its environment indicates extrinsic incoherence, and it reduces the health and viability of the organism. The following definitions can be put forward:

1) Health is an adequate level of coherence in the organism, a condition brought about and maintained by adequate access to the information that "forms" the living organism.
2) Disease is a level and form of incoherence in the organism, indicating inadequate access to in-formation. (Diseases can be classified according to the types and levels of the blockages that cause them.)
3) Diseases are pathologies of in-formation, and they are simultaneously individual and collective. They are individual when they appear to affect a single subject. This, however, is illusory. Given that organisms are dynamic elements in the biosphere, which is an intrinsically whole system, the notion of individual disease is an abstraction. Disease is a factor in the collective condition of living organisms on the planet.

The organism communicates with other organisms in its external environment consistently with its internal environment. This communication does not have definite boundaries. In the final count there is communication between every living organism and the rest of the universe. The following definitions apply:

1) The universe is a coherent system, in-formed by universal attractors.
2) The forms of life that emerge and evolve in the universe are organized along principles of complexity, coherence, resonance, and analogy, rather than of linear causality and mechanistic interaction.
3) Living systems are sensitive, complex, and whole. They are cognitive networks composed of the interaction of their parts and of the interaction of the systems themselves with their environment.

The properties of living organisms are not properties of mechanical or even biochemical systems. The most important among them are the following:

a) The properties of the organism are systemic properties; they are properties of the whole system constituted of the parts, and not the properties of the parts.

b) Interactions in the organism form a complex integral network of relationships that make up nonlocally correlated wholes; the properties of organisms are intrinsically nonlocal.

c) The organism is a whole in regard to its parts, and it is a part in regard to its environment, which is a whole constituted of its multiorganic parts. It is at the same time a part of the larger system, which is the system of life on the planet. A single synchronic scheme connects the macroscopic world of living organisms with the microscopic world of quantum particles.

d) Living organisms are nondecomposable quantum systems. The correlations that connect their elements are destroyed when their parts are separated from each other and from the systems that embed them.

e) In the mathematical formalism of quantum physics, relations between the parts of the whole system are expressed in terms of probability, and the probabilities are determined by the dynamics of the system in which they occur. Thus concepts of "entanglement" apply to living organisms, which are entangled quantum-systems entangled with other organisms in the biosphere.

The Task of Information Medicine

Information medicine upholds many of the insights that hallmark the wisdom traditions. First and foremost it "re-cognizes" the vital role of contact with nature—and hence with the universal attractors present in nature—in preserving the health and integrity of the organism.

The task of information medicine is to purposively further the preservation or restoration of coherence within the organism as well as between the organism and its environment. In traditional societies this task involved restoring contact between individual organisms or tribes and their natural environment. It was entrusted to shamans, gurus, and medicine men and women. In the modern world, the preservation and restoration of health is the task of medical doctors and other health professionals. They apply a wide range of health technologies that substitute for direct contact with nature.

However, the health-preserving and restoring effects of contact with nature, known for millennia, are irreplaceable, and they are being rediscovered. For example, the practice of "forest bathing" (*shinrin-yoku*), originating in traditional Japan, is spreading in the modern world. It is found to bring significant health benefits: lowering heart rate, reducing blood pressure, reducing stress hormone production, and improving overall well-being. Thomas Miller, editor of the Findhorn Foundation's magazine, noted: "Studies have linked even relatively small amounts of time spent in nature to better mental health, improved empathy, lengthened attention span and boosted immune system, to name only a few benefits. As more artists, writers, business people and others wake up to the benefits of 'forest bathing,' nature retreats and other ways of immersing themselves in nature, they are finding that their creativity and inspiration return."[4]

As the clinical studies cited in part two of this book testify, effective contact with natural substances that convey whole-system in-formation to the diseased organism produces remarkable healing effects. It cures, or at least increases resistance to, a wide array of autoimmune and degenerative maladies, including tumoral diseases and diseases of the cardiovascular system, the nervous system, and the digestive system. It slows the processes of cellular senescence and extends the span of healthy human life. Contact with nature furnishes the kind of guidance that the GPS (global positioning satellite) does in regard to position on the surface of the planet. This guidance is produced by nature and not by man-made technology, and it concerns the coherence—the health—of the subject and not its spatial position.

Clear and robust contact with nature is becoming difficult to achieve. This is due partly to access to nature becoming more and more remote for people in cities, and partly to the compromised quality of the nature to which people have access. As a result fewer people practice effective forest bathing, nature meditation, and other ways of entering into contact with nature. Such contact as they do achieve often proves insufficient to maintain or to regain their health.

For modern people, contact with pristine nature is becoming well-nigh impossible to achieve, and our health suffers the consequences. Not surprisingly, a significant number of compensatory measures are being developed. Modern medicine is largely focused on applying compensatory measures. Faced with a disease, or a condition of less than optimum health, physicians turn to biochemical remedies, to radiation therapy, and if necessary to surgery, to reestablish the coherence of the organism.

Modern medicine's therapeutic measures offer cures to scores of ailments, but they are not the simplest and the most effective way to preserve and restore health. A simpler and more effective way is to bring to the organism the in-formation that would in-form it in nature. The effectiveness of doing so is shown by the technical studies published in chapter two, "Information Medicine in Clinical Practice." It appears that introducing extracts from the embryo of a living organism—in this case, a Zebrafish—into a diseased or imperfectly developed organism amounts to bringing whole-system in-formation to that organism. These complex in-formation-carrying proteins exhibit remarkable healing powers: they act as stem cell differentiation stage factors (SCDSFs), reprogramming human pathological stems cells to normalcy. Reprogramming stem cells prolongs the life cycle of normal cells, reinforces the cellular and organic vitality of the organism, and slows the growth of imperfectly differentiated mutant cells.*

This in-formation-based therapy promises to be the basis of an effective, efficient, and low-cost medical technology coming online in the foreseeable future.

---

*Technical details of these healing processes are described in the scientific papers in part two, The Research.

References

1. I. K. Taimni, *Man, God and the Universe* (Madras: The Theosophical Society, 1969).
2. Das Wesen der Materie [The Nature of Matter], speech in Florence, Italy, 1944. Archiv zur Geschichte der Max Planck Gesellschaft, Abt. Va, Rep. 11 Planck, Nr. 1797.
3. B. J. Dobbs, *The Janus Faces of Genius* (Cambridge University Press, 1991).
4. Thomas Miller, Editorial in the 2018 issue dedicated to "Transforming human consciousness in everyday life," Findhorn Foundation.

CHAPTER II

Information Medicine
in Clinical Practice

The application of new paradigm medicine to clinical practice is based on the realization that the ordering-structuring factor in the universe Bohm called "in-formation," and traditional wisdom named *chi* or *qi* (or *prana* or *etheric factor*), is the key to maintaining the integrity and safeguarding the health of organisms. Clinical experience confirms the healing power of nature's in-formation, and the importance of using it in addition to, or in concert with, artificial compensatory methods.

The information contextualized by cells and cellular systems is not limited to the classically recognized biophysiological aspects of the body. The information that directs choices in the organism is supra-biological: in the last count, it is the effect of the attractor that forms and structures processes in the universe. Consequently medicine must not limit itself to the classical biochemical approaches.

It is now recognized that the causes of disease may be more than bacterial and viral: there may be deficiencies and imbalances in the organism that are not evident on the biochemical level. Subliminal psychoemotional causes could also manifest as disease. And there may be personal lifestyle and environmental factors that impact negatively on the organism. These indicate inadequate in-formation by the attractor that structures systems in space and time.

In-formation guides formative processes throughout the organism, as well as between organisms. It acts on the epigenetic system, the system that guides the activation and suppression of particular genes—which in turn regulates the functioning of the whole organism. In acting on the epigenetic system, in the final count it is the in-formation received by the organism that determines the response of the organism to the signals that reach it in its environment. In the embryo it determines the process whereby stem cells differentiate into normal cells (kidney, lung, liver, brain, and still other cells). Cellular differentiation involves a complex series of precisely sequenced steps, at the end of which every cell in the developing organism shares the same genetic code. Following cell differentiation in the embryo, the two codes remain aligned and use the same system to receive and decode messages. This enables the diverse types of cells in the embryo to "understand" each other.

Molecules and other factors of the microenvironment carry information, and cells process that information, decoding and integrating it both in regard to its form and its content. The messages elicit responses, and the responses communicate information to all the cells of the body, whether they are proximal or distant.

Communication among cells takes place when the cells are integrated in a body. Through the exchange of messages, cells constitute an integral cognitive network. This network processes information in all species of organism, including the simplest unicellular species.

As already noted, the living organism is more than the sum of its parts. The integrality of the organism ensures that the various chemical and physical-chemical reactions are not expressions of separate events but result from the fine-tuning of the organism to its intrinsic and extrinsic (internal and external) environment. It allows molecules and cells to adopt behaviors corresponding to their location within the system.

The differentiation of DNA is indispensable for the reprogramming of dysfunctional or downright malignant tumor cells toward benign behavior. To understand why, we need to look at what is happening in the body following the absorption of synthetic molecules—structures that do not exist in nature.

Let us suppose that an unnatural and for the organism unfamiliar substance produces toxic effects. Although it comes into contact with this substance for the first time, the liver, which is the organ of detoxification, is able not only to recognize the form of the message received from the unfamiliar substance but to understand the nature of its content. If the substance is toxic, cells in the liver activate one of the systems of detoxification. These activate in turn biotransformative processes that render the substance harmless. This process can take place because the differentiation of the cells that produces a new organism is a process of "cellular cognition."

Liver cells, for example, the same as other cells in the organism, have alternatives, and they make their choice among them on the basis of the signals received from the rest of the body. If these signals were not contextualized, liver cells would not process the information, and in the absence of that information they would not make the right choices; they may be killed by the toxins. Decontextualized cells die easily, while those within the organism's network are relatively robust. It is the whole system that makes cells intelligent and capable of processing information of whole-system significance. This directs molecules and cells to adopt viability-enabling behaviors.

For the organism as an integral cognitive system, it is the context that matters. The chemical and physical-chemical reactions that occur in the body are more than the expression of mechanical events governed by blind cause-effect reactions. Cells communicate with each other cognitively and adopt behaviors commensurate with the needs of the whole system. The genetic and the epigenetic systems use the same codes to process the messages.

REPROGRAMMING CANCER
STEM-LIKE CELLS

The whole organism, with all its subsystems and organs, is an integral cognitive network, and in the case of a disease such as cancer, information in that system is blocked: it does not govern the behavior of a group of malignant cells. The dialogue between the organism and that group of cells is arbitrarily uncontextualized—interrupted. The signification codes have changed; they are not the same as those in healthy, normal cells.

Cancer tumor cells organize their own behavior at the expense of the whole organism. Normally differentiated cells cooperate, and their behavior is in harmony with cells in the rest of the organism, whereas cancer cells, not being adequately in-formed, may develop malignancy and adopt counterfunctional behaviors. However, this flaw can be corrected. If the organism is given access to the in-formation that maintains or contributes to the health of the organism, it can reprogram its malfunctioning cells.

It is known that during the phase of organogenesis (when the organs are forming) in the embryo, regulatory substances are present that correct alterations caused by carcinogens in the embryo's stem cells. These substances act on the epigenetic code that regulates gene expression in the embryo. They are stem cell differentiation stage factors (SCDSFs), and they slow or stop the growth of a variety of tumors.

The behavior of tumor cells cannot be reduced to a problem of cells and genes. An explanation based solely on molecular mechanisms resulting from genetic activity and related growth factors does not clarify the nature of cancer. Cancer is a complex system where contact and communication with the flow of information among organs and systems of organs is interrupted, and the in-formation that structures and governs the living organism is inadequately accessed. As a result the health, and even the survival, of the organism is at risk.

The key discovery of information medicine is that substances produced in the dialogue between mother and embryo are effective instruments for inducing the differentiation of mutant and degenerative stem cells in the embryo. These substances are precisely tuned to the embryo's developmental stage. When extracted and applied to stem cells in other organisms, including the human, they regulate the developmental program of stem cells in those organisms. Clinical evidence shows that cells obtained at precisely selected phases of organogenesis differentiate and reprogram cancer cells in the host organism, inducing malignant cells to mutate into normal healthy cells.

The new discovery has been tested both *in vitro* (in the laboratory) and *in vivo* (under natural conditions). The testing has confirmed the discovery's effectiveness in cases of serious tumoral and degenerative diseases. Here we review some strands of the evidence, prefacing our review by a summary of the processes of embryonic differentiation.

Embryonic Differentiation Processes

Shortly after fertilization, generally in the middle-blastula-gastrula period, the processes of differentiation begin. There are basic features of the process:

- Every cell nucleus contains the complete genome produced in the fertilized egg. In molecular terms, the DNAs of all the differentiated cells are identical.
- Inactive genes in the differentiated cells are not destroyed or mutated; they retain the potential for being expressed.
- Only a small percentage of the genome is expressed in each differentiated cell, and the portion of the synthesized RNA is specific for each cell type.

Briefly, the differentiation, which leads totipotent embryonic stem cells to specialization, consists of the differential regulation of genes, restricting the genome that is expressed. The gene configurations of the cells, which arise after each stage of differentiation, differ from the progenitor cells for many expressed genes.

The differentiation of the cells is controlled by regulators: generally, these are factors that cooperate in a network that promotes and controls the differentiation of each type of cell. All cells communicate with each other through the network.

When a new organism is formed, regulation and control in each cell does not govern merely that particular cell but connects with the control system of all the cells in the organism. Systemic integration begins with embryonic development; it is what makes that development goal oriented. It takes place in all living species. Whenever a new organism is formed, its unique species code is the basis of its development.

During embryo development, cell multiplication and differentiation (or specialization) processes take place. These processes occur through a series of complex stages that take place at mind-boggling speed.

The Beginning of Cell Differentiation
in Various Types of Stem Cells

The first stage in the development of the embryo is the segmentation phase. It is a multiplicative phase, in which all the cells are totipotent, meaning that every cell can develop into a complete new organism. This phase is followed by a stage in which the first process of cellular differentiation begins; that is, the development of the blastocyst (a structure made up of an internal mass of cells that develops into an embryo from a hollow cavity surrounded by a layer of cells; in mammals, this becomes the embryonic membrane and placenta).

In this stage, not all embryonic cells are totipotent: from the cells surrounding the blastocyst, those that develop the embryonic membranes begin to differentiate. The totipotent cells of the internal mass of the blastocyst also begin to differentiate into three pluripotent stem daughter cells, which represent three primary germ cell layers; that is, the ectoderm (which develops into the skin, including mammary tissue and the nervous system), the endoderm (which will develop into the tissue of the digestive system, including the digestive glands, liver, spleen, etc.), and the mesoderm (which will develop into bones, muscle, connective tissue, and blood vessels). The cell's loss of totipotency and gain of specialized functions is the consequence of an asymmetric process of division (the mother cells on the one hand give rise to identical daughter cells and to other cells that began to differentiate into three pluripotent stem cells).

Subsequent divisions create different types of stem cells that, according to their degree of specialization, can be defined as: a) multipotent; b) oligopotent; c) progressively differentiating cells; and d) completely differentiated cells. It should be pointed out that these cells gradually acquire specialized functions and lose their ability to multiply. Indeed, completely differentiated cells cannot multiply any longer. There are cells in some tissues of the adult organisms that continue to multiply and then differentiate, such as bone marrow cells, cells that develop into blood cells, skin germ cells, and intestinal villus cells. Many cells in some tissues are in fact stem cells preserved in the adult organism.

To understand how differentiation takes place from totipotent stem cells, we have to follow the chain of events through which information is exchanged between the cells. In brief, the heart of the process is the transmission of information during the processes of replication and differentiation, making it possible for the genetic code, which is the same in all the cells of the organism, to carry out required functions in each of the specialized cells.

The Epigenetic Code

It has become clear that in addition to the genetic code, consisting of genes that codify proteins, there is also a tightly knit network of molecules and a substantial portion of DNA that perform regulatory functions. Together the network and the regulating DNA make up the "epigenetic code." This code is a precise system of regulation of gene expression active during embryonic development, and thereby determining which genes remain active and which do not; which protein products are synthesized and which are not; which molecular communication mechanisms remain operational and which do not; and in what way codifying genes interact with their products.

This is the code that makes differentiation and specialization possible as the embryo develops. This is the code that enables a totipotent embryonic stem cell to become a liver cell, kidney cell, brain cell, lung cell, and so on. Just as the conductor of an orchestra decides how a piece is to be played, so the epigenetic code decides how the codifying DNA within each cell should be read. In this way, when the differentiation process has been completed, all the differentiated cells have the same DNA as their base, but the part of active codifying genes in each differently specialized cell is specifically different and represents only a fraction of the entire DNA that it is able to codify. With the exception of very few cases, the differences between specialized cells are epigenetic and not genetic. Today the study of epigenetics is changing the face of biology. The twenty-first century will be the century of epigenetics, shifting the spotlight until now directed on the genetic code.

We are now realizing the extent of these changes: in fact, the prospects for the future in the therapeutic field are likely to stem from this branch of research rather than from genetics, where results linked to genetic manipulation are ethically questionable.

Let us at this point examine the various stages of epigenetic regulation to which totipotent embryonic stem cells are subject until they become fully differentiated cells. As already mentioned, in a multicellular organism with specialized cells and tissue, each cell possesses all the genes of that organism. The difference between specialized cells is due to the specific activity of the genes that continue to function even after the specific and selective silencing to which many of them are subject during the differentiation of the embryonic cell. This process of differentiation is very precise and finely tuned. So during this process certain proteins must therefore be synthesized at the right moment and in the right cell: gene expression in this way is strictly controlled and the possibility of error is very low. Unlike DNA replication, which generally in each cell is regulated according to the "all or nothing" principle, gene expression is a highly selective process.

Chromatin Remodeling

One of the first places in which the regulatory process occurs is at chromatin level, which is the material contained in the cell nucleus and composed of dense DNA wrapped around a center made up of proteins called histones, which play an important role in compacting nucleic acid.

Just under two DNA folds, composed of 146 nucleotides, wrap around a center composed of eight histones to form a structure that resembles a pearl in a necklace and is called a "nucleosoma." With the help of other histone proteins that link the centers of the various nucleosomes with the DNA interposed between them, the string of nucleosomes folds and becomes a chromatin fiber that is further compacted. The degree of chromatin density impacts accessibility to important factors for the transcription of the genes contained therein. The more compact the chromatin, the less accessible the transcription factors. One way to keep a gene from transcribing is through methylation whereby a group of CH_3 is attached to some of cells' bases. In this case the DNA sequence is not modified, but the chromatin is compacted, thereby determining the probability of transcription, which at this point is lower. Conversely, adding acetylic groups (C_2H_5) to certain amino-acids of histones usually leads to a looser chromatin structure, thereby increasing the likelihood of transcription. Removing the acetylic groups from the histone proteins, like methylating their amino acids, renders the chromatin denser and does not allow the DNA to be transcribed. The remodeling of the chromatin can involve an entire chromosome; for example, one of the X chromosomes determining gender. It is widely known that normal female mammals have two X chromosomes while normal male mammals have an X chromosome and a Y chromosome. Between males and females there is a sizable difference in terms of the "dosage" of genes linked to the X chromosome. In other words, each cell of a female has two copies of genes present in the X chromosome and can potentially produce twice the proteins codified by these genes compared to male cells. This does not occur because during cell differentiation one of the two maternal X chromosomes is methylated and its chromatin is condensed in such a way that the DNA sequences become inaccessible to the transcription molecular machinery.

Transcriptional and Post-Transcriptional Regulation

Transcription is the first step of gene expression, in which a particular segment of DNA is copied into RNA. Both DNA and RNA are nucleic acids, which use base pairs of nucleotides as a complementary language. The transcription machinery is highly complex and is made up of proteins called *transcription factors,* which are necessary to an enzyme called RNA *polymerases* to form a complex that determines the starting point of transcription. This complex binds to a DNA sequence called a *promoter* and is the region where the transcription of the codifying region of the gene is promoted. At the opposite end of this ladder is a region of the DNA called *terminator,* the point at which transcription is terminated. In this way there are precise start and stop signals built into the transcription of DNA into RNA.

At the transcriptional level there are many regulatory events that significantly change gene expression. Regulating regions have been recently discovered that are immediately grouped at the origin of the promoter. Various regulating proteins can link up to these regions and can activate transcription. Far from the promoter we find intensifying sequences (intensifiers). These sequences bind activating proteins and this greatly stimulates the transcription complex.

In DNA, there are also negative regulating regions, silencing sequences, which have an effect opposite to that of the intensifiers. *Silencers* arrest transcription and link the proteins called *suppressors.* In some cases, gene expression is regulated by the movement of a gene to a new position on the chromosome. As a result, the DNA is rearranged. This is important, among other things, for producing highly variable proteins, such as those that make up the repertoire of human antibodies.

Rearrangement is also important in determining certain forms of cancer in which inactive genes can move next to active promoters.

Another type of regulation is known as "genetic amplification." This occurs, for example, in the mature egg cells of amphibians and fishes. After fertilization, a trillion ribosomes are necessary for protein synthesis. Cells that differentiate into egg cells initially contain less than one thousand copies of genes that codify for the ribosomal RNA. It would take about fifty years to synthesize all this RNA. Egg cells have solved this problem by selectively increasing the group of genes for ribosomal RNA, thereby hugely increasing the quantity. In fact this group of genes rises from 0.2% to 68% of total codifying DNA. These million copies that transcribe very quickly synthesize in just a few days the trillion ribosomes needed for the next protein synthesis.

In terms of post-transcriptional regulation processes, there is an extremely important mechanism in evolved organisms, which is linked to a process known as "alternative RNA splicing." In the DNA, codifying sequences, called *exons*, are next to noncodifying sequences, known as *introns*. Transcribed introns appear in the primary RNA transcriptions called *pre-mRNA*, which undergo a splicing process before arriving in the cytoplasm in large complexes of RNA and proteins called *spliceosomes* in which the introns of primary transcription of the RNA are eliminated and the exons are grouped together. This messenger RNA (mature mRNA) is translated into polypeptides (proteins). Splicing is often much more complex, as it can make many different cuts that are able to give rise to multiple messenger RNA and consequently to differing protein.

Another post-transcriptional regulatory event is the one linked to RNA editing, which takes place essentially either by inserting new nucleotides into the mRNA or by chemically modifying a nucleotide. In both cases the synthesized protein is modified. Even the survival time of messenger RNA in the cytoplasm undergoes post-transcriptional regulation. The less time mRNA spends in the cytoplasm, the fewer the codified proteins synthesized by mRNA.

Finally, regulation mechanisms that are important in terms of transcription and in terms of post-transcription, but also in terms of translation of the proteins, are those linked to the action of RNA regulators. In particular, the so-called micro RNAs (miRNAs) have great importance, because they recognize the sequence of target messenger RNAs and mate with them, thereby keeping them from being translated into proteins. In this case, we can speak of translational regulation. MiRNAs are involved in cell differentiation, and they have a significant impact on the regulation of gene expression and therefore on the development of an organism. Studies in which a part of the machinery of miRNA processing was destroyed have shown that an organism cannot survive without the regulator role that miRNA plays. Another bizarre trait of these small RNAs is their ability to move to other cells, even different types, and thus cause genetic silencing from a distance.

Translational and Post-Translational Regulation

Having addressed above how specific microRNA uses the translational regulation mechanism to block the translation of specific mRNA (which obviously prevents the corresponding proteins from being synthesized), we are now focusing on translational regulation events. These latter events are often connected to the concentration of specific proteins that need to be synthesized. When their concentration is low, the speed at which messenger RNA already present in the cytoplasm translates them increases. Inversely, when their concentration is high, translation slows down.

Lastly, proteins can be regulated after they have been synthesized. An important post-translational regulation event is tied to the control of survival time of proteins within the cell itself. It is well known how some proteins involved in cellular division, like cyclins, are hydrolyzed at just the right moment so that sequencing can develop correctly over time. In many instances a protein that is to be degraded is linked to a polypeptide chain composed of seventy-six amino acids called *ubiquitin* (so-called because it is ubiquitous). This complex in turn binds to another large complex made up of a dozen polypeptides called *proteasomes,* which make up a sort of molecular destruction chamber in which the degrading protein is destroyed. The fact that so many proteins are concentrated within the cell is not determined by the differing speeds of transcription of the genes, but rather by how fast proteasomes destroy the molecules.

In short, cellular differentiation consists of a differential, specific, and selective gene regulation process that essentially restricts the expressed genome. A cell's gene expression after each stage of differentiation is different from the progenitor cell in regard to hundreds of expressed genes. This is possible, as we mentioned earlier, because a gene, which in the past was thought to be the control center independent and autonomous from protein synthesis, in actual fact is directly and indirectly controlled by a regulation network and by synthesized proteins. In the embryo, the intense and extended interaction between the nucleus and the cytoplasm and the cytoplasm and the microenvironment is a prime example of complexity. An embryo under development and differentiation is an excellent example of what complexity researchers have termed "a complex adaptive system."

The above system is made up of a network of multiple cells that act in parallel and have differing levels of organization. They are constantly subjected to revision and control. In addition, this system has an implicit prediction written in its genetic code and in the epigenetic regulatory events. Lastly, the system is in continuous transition and changes constantly. In this way, the totipotent stem cells that are produced first give rise to pluripotent stem cells, then to multipotent stem cells, and then oligopotent cells, until a new organism is formed. At this point, it is clear that stem cell differentiation stage factors (SCDSFs) present at the different stages of cell differentiation represent the epigenetic code, the system that can transmit whole-system information—that is, "in-formation" to the organism. This has remarkable healing properties.

Studies on the functioning of the epigenetic code revealed that this code is present in its totality and with all its various functions the moment life appears in the embryo.

This code—that is the "in-formation" of the embryo—can be

studied and understood in its global functions, even if divided into the various stages of differentiation. When all of the code, that is, the entire "in-formation" that regulates the genes of all the cells that make up the organism, is before us, we have what has been called the *Code of Life.*

The possibility of studying the epigenetic code in its entirety exists only in the embryo, and only in the period of organogenesis, when starting from a single totipotent stem cell, through various stages that form all the types of stem cells: pluripotent, multipotent, oligopotent, definitively differentiating cells, and finally complete differentiated cells.

When organogenesis is over, it is no longer possible to study the entire epigenetic code in its various functions. This is because, when organogenesis is completed, the epigenetic code subdivides in the various organs and tissues, and in every organ serves to control and regulate the gene expression of the cells. At that point, it is no longer possible to study all the various functions of the Code of Life.

However, research prior to the completion of organogenesis permits studying the entire Code of Life. This research allowed us to discover how to prolong the life span and to stop the senescence of cells, how to regenerate the tissues and reinforce the cellular and organic vitality of the organism, how to slow the growth of imperfectly differentiated cells, and how to induce altered stem cells to differentiate into normal cells—or undergo programmed cell death.

REVIEW OF THE
EXPERIMENTAL EVIDENCE

Here we record various experiments with stem cell differentiation stage factors (SCDSFs). These factors are accessible at different stages of the differentiation of the cells of the embryo of the Zebrafish. The choice of the tiny Zebrafish may appear arbitrary, but it has sound reasons: notwithstanding their size and relative simplicity, Zebrafish have very largely the same proteins as humans, and access to their genetic material is simple and safe. In addition, it is easy to discover the exact time of the fertilization of Zebrafish eggs. This is important for standardizing the experiments.

Results of the Experiment In Vitro

Six different human tumor lines (including a malignant brain tumor, primary liver tumor, colon and breast cancer, kidney tumor, and acute lymphoblastic leukemia) have been treated with factors obtained from Zebrafish embryos in four different developmental stages: a) morula stage, characterized by cell-multiplicatory events only, and therefore constituted of totipotent embryonic stem cells; b) medium-blastula-gastrula stage, where the totipotent embryo stem cells differentiate into pluripotent stem cells; c) the five somite stage; and d) the twenty somite stage, where important differentiation events of the intermediate and final embryo differentiation process take place.

All cell lines have shown a significant slowdown in growth when treated with factors drawn during the above-mentioned cell-differentiation stages, with inhibition percentages ranging from 73 percent of the malignant brain tumor to 26 percent of the melanoma. No effects have been registered with factors extracted in the morula stage, except for a weak tumoral growth.[1]

The above data confirms the hypothesis that during the stages of differentiation, factors are present in the embryo that address tumoral cells and reorient them toward the normal path. These factors appear in the very first phases of differentiation, and they are absent in stages of mere multiplication.

Several studies were carried out in order to understand which molecular events are involved in the tumor-growth inhibition mechanism. It appears that molecules that have a fundamental role in the cellular cycle regulation process, such as p53 and pRb, are involved through transcriptional and post-translational regulation events. More precisely, a p53 transcriptional regulation (meaning the activation of the tumor-suppressing gene with the synthesis of p53 protein) was obtained, highlighted by a considerable increase of the p53 protein's concentration in the cells of some tumor lines, such as melanoma and brain tumor. This has been measured through the quantitative as well as the immune-histochemical method, after treatment with the cell-differentiation factors.[2]

The slowdown of tumor growth on other tumor lines, such as kidney cancer, is due to the post-translational regulation of a protein (pRb), which is named *restriction factor of cell cycle*—this indicates the regulation of the already translated protein of the retinoblastoma—and leads to a change in the relation between the protein's phosphorylated and non-phosphorylated shape.[3] It is well known that the non-phosphorylated shape stops the cellular cycle, preventing the transcription of the E2F-1 gene. The latter is facilitated when the protein is phosphorylated.

Finally, programmed cell-death events (apoptosis) as well as cell-differentiation events were studied, in order to understand the consequences of the tumor-cell regulation cycle by the differentiation factors. The analysis was carried out on colon adenocarcinoma cells, demonstrating the activation of an apoptotic pathway as well as a cell-differentiation pathway. Within a culture of colon tumor cells, there was a significant increase in apoptosis, as well as in the concentration of cell-differentiation markers.[4] Therefore, the molecular mechanisms at the basis of the slowdown of tumor growth due to treatment with SCDSFs can be summed up as follows: cessation of the cell cycle in accordance with the type of tumor, genetic damage repair, and cell re-differentiation—or the apoptosis (death) of the tumor cells (if repair is no longer possible).

Clinical Results

Results from Clinical Trials on Intermediate-Advanced Hepatocellular Carcinoma (HCC)

A randomized controlled trial was conducted from January 1, 2001, to April 31, 2004, on 179 patients affected by HCC in the intermediate-advanced stage, for which no further treatment was possible, such as liver resection or transplantation, chemo-embolization, ablation with radiofrequency, or other type of treatments. A product was administered fine-tuned on the basis of the above studies. The dosage was thirty sublingual drops three times a day. (The sublingual solution was chosen because the active fraction is composed of low molecular weight proteins and nucleic acids.)

Objective tumor response and median overall survival and performance status have been evaluated. Results show that 19.8 percent of the patients experienced a regression and 16 percent of the patients experienced stabilization with an overall survival after forty months of more than 60 percent of the patients who responded, compared with 10 percent of the nonresponding patients.

A wide improvement of performance status has been registered in a great majority of patients (82.6 percent), including in those who are in the progressive phase of the disease.[5] A recent study of reprogramming normal and cancerous stem cells confirms the role of SCDSFs in producing a complete response in 13.1 percent patients experiencing primitive, intermediate, or advanced liver cancer.[6]

Results of Experiments on Neurodegenerative Diseases

It has been shown that the completeness of the information and the redundancy of factors of the epigenetic code are able to significantly prevent the degeneration of the nervous cells; for example, the cells of the hippocampus. This happens because initially the redundancy of all the factors present from the beginning of the differentiation process first expands the number of stem cells and then differentiates them in the specific tissue. In other words, what we have understood by conducting the experiments on the hippocampal cells, the cells that first undergo neurodegeneration in Alzheimer's disease, is that if we want to prevent the degeneration of these cells, we must exactly simulate the program that life adopts to self-organize and realize itself.

First we must, as already mentioned above, administer the substances that keep the stem genes turned on, allowing the survival of the few stem cells left active in the brain of an Alzheimer patient and therefore keeping their number intact, but then we must administer the substances that are able to differentiate stem cells in specific nervous cells. To obtain this result, we must exactly simulate the process that originates life and administer all the factors that are able to make the whole process of the cells perform.

With various collaborators we are now studying how the different specific molecules that make up the epigenetic code are able to repair the tissues and therefore can be used in regenerative medicine, in particular in pathologies where stem cell transplantation is required. These epigenetic regulators can in fact enhance the positive effects related to stem cell transplantation and in the future replace the same transplant, considering that it has been shown that the beneficial effects due to the stem cell transplantation are not due to the transplanted cells, but to the factors that they produce. And the factors that they produce are the same factors which constitute the epigenetic code.[7]

Results of Clinical Studies on Psoriasis

Two clinical trials[8,9] were conducted to evaluate the efficacy of a topical formulation of Zebrafish embryo extracts with Boswellia serrata, 18-beta glycyrrhetinic acid, Zanthoxylum alatum, 7-deidrocolesterolo, and vitamin E in cases of psoriasis. Results show a very high clinical objective improvement, with a reduction of keratosis and itch after 20 to 30 days from the beginning of the treatment.

Results of Anti-Aging Studies

Studies by Biava et al. on antiaging processes demonstrate that the very early stage of cell differentiation is able to activate the same genes that Shinya Yamanaka introduced with a retrovirus in a completely differentiated cell, reprogramming it into so-called induced pluripotent stem cells, an accomplishment for which he received the 2012 Nobel Prize in Physiology and Medicine. Biava and collaborators are able to activate the same genes without physical manipulation, on the basis of epigenetic "in-formational" regulation. In this case, the cells maintain their cyclicity, whereas in the case of the physical manipulation of the DNA, as in the experiments of Yamanaka, the cells lose their cyclicity. This is important, because in in-formational regulation the cells maintain their physiological characteristics, whereas those characteristics are lost in DNA manipulation.

The above experiments demonstrate that one can maintain not only the functions of the genes that halt the sectioning of telomeres, thereby increasing the cell's life span, but also activate other genes that stop the senescence of the cells. In this way, the cells increase not only their life span, but maintain themselves in a youthful stage (see the paper included in part two: The Research: "Stem Cell Differentiation Stage Factors from Zebrafish Embryo: A Novel Strategy to Modulate the Fate of Normal and Pathological Human (Stem) Cells)."

CONCLUSIONS BASED ON THE EXPERIMENTS

The use of stem cell differentiation stage factors in anticancer therapy enabled the development of a new model of cancer.[10] In that model, cancer cells are undifferentiated cells, in which mutation or epigenetic alterations are present that block the cells in a multiplication phase between two stages of differentiation.

Therefore cancer cells can be defined as "altered stem cells," in which mutations of DNA or epigenetic alterations are present. These cells, according to their degree of malignancy, are blocked at a particular phase of their development. In support of this model we should note that in tumors with an elevated degree of malignancy, such as acute lymphoblastic and myeloid leukemia, multipotent altered stem cells are present, whereas in tumors with lower malignancy, such as chronic lymphocytic leukemia, incompletely differentiated cells are present, which can then progress toward further differentiation.

This model is supported by the finding that cancer cells and stem cells have common characteristics. The common elements are the presence of oncofetal antigens, maintained during phylogenesis,[11] and the specific receptor on the cellular membrane on which the differentiation factors appear to act. As already mentioned, such factors activate metabolic pathways of cellular differentiation, and these pathways lead the cells to differentiate or to die (enter apoptosis). The latter is the usual occurrence in the embryo, where there are many apoptotic pathways.

The problem of cancer stem-like cells is twofold: not only do they present the genetic mutations that (so far as is known) are at the origin of malignancy, but they also manifest important modifications of the epigenetic code. The gene configuration and the metabolism of cancer cells are similar to those in stem cells: both have active proto-oncogenes, both produce embryonic growth factors, and in addition tumor cells present oncofetal antigens expressed by normal stem cells. Both work with an anaerobic metabolism. The difference between them is that tumoral cells, in contrast with normal stem cells, are not able to complete their development and to differentiate, having lost the necessary in-formation in the alteration of their epigenetic code. The correction of this condition calls for the use of the differentiation factors that transform cancer cells into normal cells.

DNA is responsible, via RNA, for the translation of proteins, so that the transcription factors, the microRNAs and the translational and post-translational factors play a fundamental role in the regulation of the genetic code, and thus in the regulation of the life cycle of cells. The epigenetic code can differentiate and regulate normal stem cells as well as cancer stem-like cells, deactivating genes that govern cancer stem-like cells and activating the pathways of differentiation that lead to normal cells.

The results reported here have been confirmed by research at the Children's Hospital of Chicago. In particular, research confirmed that malignant melanoma reverts to a normal phenotype when it is in the environment of a Zebrafish embryo. At the same time, a growing body of studies highlighted that tumor malignancy is linked to the presence of tumoral stem cells,[12] and these appear resistant to conventional therapy, such as chemo- and radiotherapy. In the last few years, scientific studies in this area have been so numerous that it is nearly impossible to take all of them into account. Here we mention only the research that demonstrates the presence of tumoral stem cells in breast cancer,[13] lung cancer,[14,15,16,17] prostate cancer,[18,19] ovary cancer,[20,21,22,23] liver cancer,[24,25,26,27,28,29] stomach cancer,[30,31,32,33,34] colon cancer,[35,36,37,38] pancreas cancer,[39,40,41] head and neck cancer,[42,43,44,45] glioblastoma.[46,47,48] It is known that malignancy in many hematological tumoral diseases is due to the presence of stem cells.

The results of antiaging treatments and the prevention of neurodegenerative disorders point to the same processes: the differentiation factors are epigenetic regulators with different specific functions. They are like an orchestra that can interpret different symphonies. The use of epigenetic regulation factors can be widely applied in the prevention and treatment of degenerative diseases, not only of the nervous system but also of the cardiovascular-osteoarticular system, diabetes, and others. They are also antiaging factors, improving the overall state of health of the elderly.

Noteworthy is that for the in-formation carried by the regulating factors to be effective, it must be transferred not in individual bits, but in precise instruction packages. In fact, every cell-differentiation process occurs only if multiple genes (rather than a single gene) are simultaneously addressed and regulated. Life is organized on the basis of in-formation programs that provide integral and precise instruction packages: these packages act as integral wholes. If they are fragmented, they lose their effectiveness. Experiments with cellular differentiation factors confirm that the organism is a unitary mind-body system.

Information is crucial to the processes of this integral body-mind system; its regulation is in the form of factors of information. This information is the "in-formation" that "forms" evolutionary processes in the universe. It is the manifest effect of a universal attractor that codes complex and coherent systems for integrality and health. For a human organism maintaining and, if needed, restoring health calls for effective contact with this attractor, ensuring the effective reception of the in-formation that orients living systems toward health and normalcy. Stem cell differentiation stage factors (SCDSFs) are factors of information that ensure such contact for systems suffering from diseases due to imperfect forms of cellular differentiation.

ADDENDUM: DECLARATION OF A COMMITTEE OF ONCOLOGISTS

....

Stem Cell Differentiation Factors as Integrative Treatments in Oncology: Their Role in Increasing the Efficacy of Chemotherapy and in Reducing its Adverse Effects

Edited by Michele Carruba, Chairman of the Scientific Committee, Director of the Department of Pharmacology of the University of Milan

Parallel to the sequencing of the genetic code, another area of research, that of epigenetics, emerged. There are therefore two types of code: the genetic and the epigenetic code that is above the genetic code and regulates its functioning. In the field of epigenetic approaches, and in particular in the field of cancer, the research on the reprogramming of tumor stem cells with embryo differentiation factors has been consolidating for several years. In fact, it has been shown that the differentiation factors of stem cells extracted from a Zebrafish egg, which has over 90 percent of common proteins with human ones, are able to normalize the cell cycle of cancerous cells.

These are the same mechanisms that in nature are active during the phases of organogenesis, when all the stem cell differentiation processes that lead to the formation of tissues and organs take place. In these phases, where there is a high risk of developing errors in replication, differentiation factors play an important role in correcting those cells that are making mistakes. Reconfirmation of this mechanism occurred when cancer cells were implanted into an embryo during the organogenesis phase: differentiated and apoptotic processes were observed on the implanted tumor cells. On the contrary, when tumor cells were implanted into an embryo *after* the organogenesis phase, they continued to proliferate. One can therefore talk of epigenetic reprogramming of diseased cells through the integration of those peptides that are able to restore the cell within its normal physiology.

These researches, begun in the late 1980s by Biava et al.[49] were then developed by the Children's Hospital in Chicago, Northwestern University, La Sapienza University of Rome, and other institutions. It emerges that differentiation factors are able, in association with standard chemotherapy treatments, to slow and often block the cell cycle of tumor cells, either by activating in a transcriptional way the p53 oncorepressor gene, or by regulating in a post-translational way the protein of retinoblastoma (pRb), which also has a block cell cycle activity. At the same time, a series of regulating gene cascades are also activated by the same differentiation factors as they attempt to repair cellular damage at the origin of malignancy: if the alterations are not too serious, they are effectively repaired; if mutations are too serious and are not repaired, the genes of programmed cell death (apoptosis) are activated and the cancerous cells die.

In fact, after treatment with stem cell differentiation factors, tumor cells leave the cellular multiplication cycle. A number of important researches on the synergy between chemotherapeutic agents and differentiation factors have already been carried out in 2011. For example, research conducted at Current Pharmaceutical Biotechnology at La Sapienza University in Rome obtained in vitro the slowdown of growth of CaCo2 colon cancer cells: a 35 percent slowdown was obtained by treatment with Fluorouracil alone, while a 98 percent slowdown was obtained with the simultaneous administration of 5-Fluorouracil and differentiation factors. Richard Ablin (PSA discoverer) reported in an article published in 2014 a greatly beneficial effect on the synergy between differentiation factors and surgical ablation or other traditional prostate cancer treatments. Stem cell differentiation factors also demonstrated improved performance and quality of life in 82 percent of patients treated; it also reduced adverse side effects of chemotherapy.

The figures on pages 42–49 are the main images related to the different studies carried out on embryo differentiation factors. The state of the art of research includes both in vitro work on molecular dynamics involving stem differentiation factors and in vivo work on mice and on humans. It remains necessary to implement in vivo research, especially the clinical kind. Specifically, studies have been conducted on the following aspects:

- Downloading and/or blocking of the cell cycle
- Activating in a transcriptional way the oncosupressor gene p53
- Regulating in a post-translational way the retinoblastoma protein (pRb)
- Slowing the growth of tumor cell lines
- Animal studies
- Protein analysis of Zebrafish egg extract
- Clinical study of 200 patients to evaluate possible side effects
- Randomized clinical study in 179 patients with intermediate or advanced hepatocarcinoma

Activation of Oncosuppressor p53

It has been shown that in the embryonic microenvironment there are factors that regulate the expression of the p53 oncorepressor, activating it, and post-translationally pRb. In fact, with the differentiation of stem cell differentiating factors of different tumor lines, a block of cell cycle was observed in G1-S phase.

Through cytofluorometry and immunohistochemistry, a significant increase in the concentration of p53 protein has been demonstrated in specific lines of cellular tumor lines such as multiform glioblastoma, melanoma, and hepatocarcinoma treated with stem differentiation

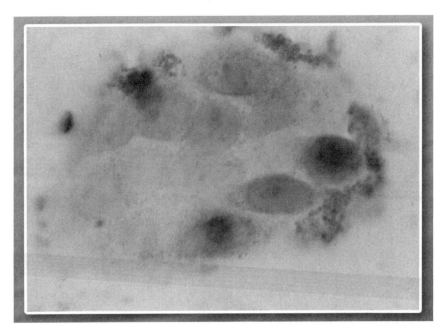

Fig. 2.1. Concentration of p53 protein (dark colored) in glioblastoma cells
before the treatment with SCDSFs

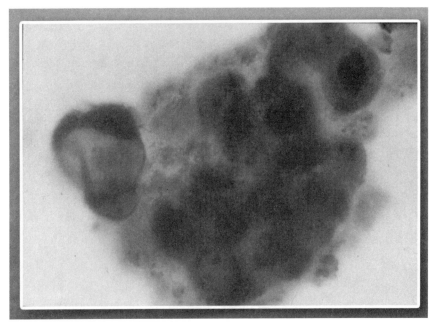

Fig. 2.2. Concentration of p53 protein (dark colored) in glioblastoma cells
after the treatment with SCDSFs

factors. This increase is a consequence of the transcriptional regulation of the p53 oncosupressor gene. The two images on page 42 show the concentration of the p53 protein before and after the treatment.[50]

Post-Translational Regulation of the
Retinoblastoma Protein

By treating cancer cell lines such as those of kidney adenocarcinoma, a post-translational regulation of retinoblastoma protein (pRb) was observed, known for its cell cycle block function. This adjustment involves modification of the relationship between the phosphorylated

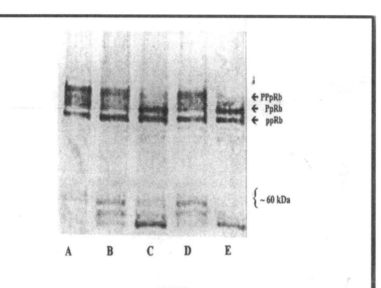

Immunostaining of whole ACHN cell lysates with α-pRb antibody after fractionation of proteins on a 5% SDS-PAGE and Western Blotting. A: untreated cells. B: 24-hours treated cells with 3 μg of extract. C: 48-hours treated cells with 3 μg of extract. D: 24-hours treated cells with 15 μg of extract. E: 48-hours treated cells with 15 μg of extract.

PPpRb: hyperphosphorylated pRb. PpRb: phosphorylated pRb. ppRb: hypophosphorylated pRb

Fig. 2.3. Post-translational modification of the retinoblastoma protein (pRb) induced by in vitro administration of Zebrafish embryonic extracts on human kidney adenocarcinoma cell line

form and the nonphosphorylated form of the pRb protein in favor of the nonphosphorylated form. This form blocks the cell cycle, stopping the transcription of the E2F-1 gene.[51]

Slow-down of the Growth of Tumor Cell Lines

These blocking mechanisms of the cell cycle have been observed in several tumor cell lines. Specifically, tumor cell lines were investigated of: glioblastoma, melanoma, breast cancer, lymphoblastic leukemia, and kidney adenocarcinoma. The following figures illustrate the cell proliferation curves of different human tumor lines after in vitro treatment with Zebrafish embryonic extracts.[52]

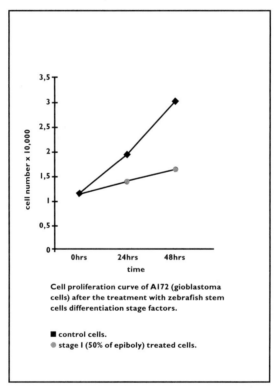

Cell proliferation curve of A172 (gioblastoma cells) after the treatment with zebrafish stem cells differentiation stage factors.

■ control cells.
● stage I (50% of epiboly) treated cells.

Fig. 2.4. Glioblastoma

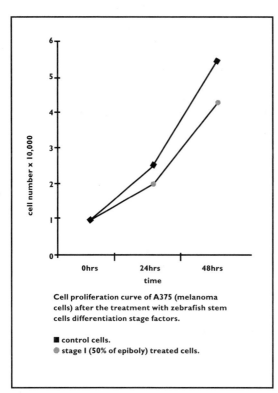

Fig. 2.5. Melanoma

Cell proliferation curve of A375 (melanoma cells) after the treatment with zebrafish stem cells differentiation stage factors.

■ control cells.
● stage I (50% of epiboly) treated cells.

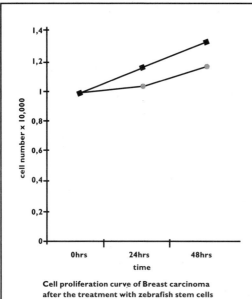

Fig. 2.6. Breast cancer

Cell proliferation curve of Breast carcinoma after the treatment with zebrafish stem cells differentiation stage factors.

■ control cells.
● stage I (50% of epiboly) treated cells.

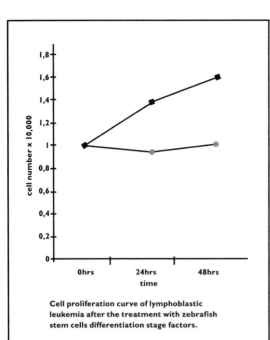

Fig. 2.7. Acute lymphoblastic leukemia

Cell proliferation curve of lymphoblastic leukemia after the treatment with zebrafish stem cells differentiation stage factors.

■ **control cells.**
● **stage I (50% of epiboly) treated cells.**

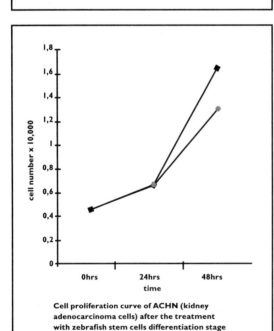

Fig. 2.8. Kidney adenocarcinoma

Cell proliferation curve of ACHN (kidney adenocarcinoma cells) after the treatment with zebrafish stem cells differentiation stage factors.

■ **control cells.**
● **stage I (50% of epiboly) treated cells.**

Animal Studies

The effects of stem differentiation factors on inhibition of tumor growth were in vivo tested on females of singular C57BL / 6 mice from the weight of 18 to 20 grams to which a subcutaneous Lewis primary carcinoma injection was performed. Therefore, both the size of the primary tumor and the survival time of the mice have been evaluated. In terms of development of the primary tumor, an extremely significant difference (P<0.001) was observed between treated and control mice (fig. 2.9) and thus also with regard to the survival ratio, always in favor of the treated mouse.[53]

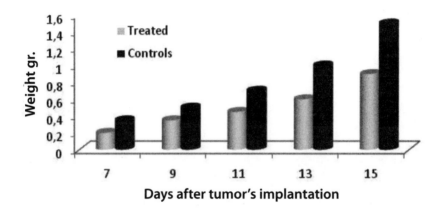

Fig. 2.9. The effects of stem differentiation factors on inhibition of tumor growth

Protein Analysis of Zebrafish Egg Extract

A protein analysis of embryonic extract from Zebrafish eggs was performed. A suspension of the glycerol-alcohol solution was analyzed with monodimensional gel electrophoresis (SDS-PAGE). As shown in figure 2.10, in all five phases extracted, they can be distinguished by their molecular weight by three major groups: over 45 kDa, about 25 to 35 kDa and below 20 kDa. In any case, the relative amount of protein is different in the five-stage samples.

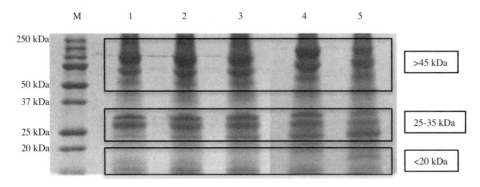

Fig. 2.10. Protein analysis of embryonic extract from Zebrafish eggs: suspension of the glycerol-alcohol solution analyzed with monodimensional gel electrophoresis (SDS-PAGE)

Below is the list of proteins that have been identified by Biava et al. with mass spectrometry analysis (see page 97). The asterisk (*) lists the proteins that have never before been described in the Zebrafish embryo.

Table 1
List of proteins identified using the nano LC-ESI-Q-TOF in Zebrafish embryo at middle-blastula-gastrula stage

Accession	Protein Name	Score	Molecular Weight	pI calculated	Sequence coverage
gi|166795887	vitellogenin 1 precursor	1108	150308	8,68	19
gi|94733730	vitellogenin 1	1039	149825	8,74	21
gi|94733733	novel protein similar to vitellogenin 1 (vg1)	913	149828	8,92	19
gi|94733734	novel protein similar to vitellogenin 1 (vg1)	835	150550	8,83	16
gi|145337918	Vtg1 protein	780	116965	9,07	18
gi|94733731	novel protein similar to vitellogenin 1 (vg1)	762	149911	8,84	19
gi|94732723	novel protein similar to vitellogenin 1 (vg1)	745	147826	8,73	17
gi|159155252*	Zgc:136383 protein	720	124413	8,78	17
gi|68448530	vitellogenin 5	559	149609	8,77	13
gi|92097636	Zgc:136383	402	28924	9,33	36
gi|63100501	Vtg1 protein	345	36580	9,23	28
gi|57864789	vitellogenin 7	341	24490	8,37	40
gi|57864783	vitellogenin 4	334	31304	9,48	27
gi|113678458	vitellogenin 2 isoform 1 precursor	323	181208	8,70	11
gi|125857991	Zgc:136383 protein	171	149328	8,93	9
gi|15209312*	procollagen type I alpha 2 chain	169	147826	9,35	4
gi|57864779	vitellogenin 2	122	69906	7,84	8
gi|11118642	vitellogenin 3 precursor	117	140477	6,92	2
gi|303227889	vitellogenin 6	73	151677	8,84	4

Accession	Protein Name	Score	Molecular Weight	pI calculated	Sequence coverage
gi|13242157 *	egg envelope protein ZP2 variant A	71	48194	6,04	5
gi|6644111 *	nucleoside diphosphate kinase-Z1	69	17397	7,77	14
gi|18859071*	nucleoside diphosphate kinase 3	69	19558	7,68	7
gi|126632622*	novel prot. cont. a galactose binding lectin domain	67	19245	9,33	13
gi|66773080 *	mitochondrial ATP synthase beta subunit-like	66	55080	5,25	4
gi|38541767*	Ppia protein	60	19745	9,30	13
gi|1865782	HSC70 protein	58	71473	5,18	2
gi|28279108	heat shock protein 8	58	71382	5,32	4
gi|41152402*	histone H2B 3	49	13940	10,31	11
gi|41393113*	collagen, type I, alpha 1b precursor	46	137815	5,39	4
gi|94732492 *	ras homolog gene family, member F	46	24035	9,00	6
gi|47778620 *	tryptophan hydroxylase D2	45	55686	6,56	1
gi|68448517 *	zona pellucida glycoprotein 3.2 precursor	44	47365	4,92	2
gi|326677766 *	PREDICTED: RIMS-binding protein 2-like	41	138659	5,86	0
gi|112419298	Vtg3 protein	40	60622	6,32	2
gi|54400406 *	glutaredoxin 3	39	36541	5,18	11
gi|41152400*	peptidylprolyl isomerase A, like	37	17763	8,26	7

Ions score is -10*Log(P), where P is the probability that the observed match is a random event.
Individual ions scores > 36 indicate identity or extensive homology (p<0.05).
Protein scores are derived from ions scores as a non-probabilistic basis for ranking protein hits.

Clinical Studies

Two clinical studies have been carried out, first to check the safety and then the effectiveness of integration of standard chemotherapy treatments with stem differentiation factors. A first study was conducted on 200 patients, including 60 with advanced breast cancer, to evaluate possible side effects: for this reason no control group was foreseen. The protocol included administering patients 1 ml three times a day as sublingual drops containing 3 microgram/ml staminal differentiation factors. After three years of treatment, no adverse events were reported in any of the 200 patients treated. In addition, 80 percent of these patients showed an improvement in the performance status, evaluated with the E.C.O.G scale: generally, the status shifted from a 4 to 3 state to one of 2 or 1. In the 60 breast cancer patients there were also four cases of partial regression and 70 percent of survival after three years.

The second study of embryonic differentiation factors with

anticancer properties produced preliminary clinical results in the therapy for advanced tumors. A randomized clinical trial was performed on 179 patients with intermediate or advanced hepatocarcinoma. The results showed a statistically significant difference between the group treated with the synergy of differentiation factors and standard treatments and the control group (P = 0.03), a difference in favor of the group treated with integration. There was 19.8 percent of regression (2.5 percent of which was total regression) and 16 percent disease stabilization.[54]

Conclusions of the Committee of Oncologists

The committee met to evaluate the scientific soundness of the reported investigations, and it confirmed the importance of this course of study and encouraged at the university level the development of further research both on an in vivo model and at a clinical level. There is also the possibility of developing food supplements that inspire these researches to provide physicians with a valuable support to integrate many of the differentiation factors described in the text. Such solutions are to be understood only as integration into standard therapies, and it is hoped that they can be validated in advance by appropriate clinical trials.

References

1. Biava, P.M.; Bonsignorio, D.; Hoxa, M. Cell proliferation curves of different human tumor lines after in vitro treatment with aafish embryonic extracts. *J. Tumor Marker Oncol.*, 2001, *16*(3), 195–202.

2. Biava, P.M.; Carluccio, A. Activation of anti-oncogene p53 produced by embryonic extracts in vitro tumor cells. *J. Tumor Marker Oncol.*, 1977, *12*(4), 9–15.

3. Biava, P.M.; Bonsignorio, D.; Hoxa, M.; Impagliazzo, M.; Facco, R.; Ielapi, T.; Frati, L.; Bizzarri, M. Post-translational modification of the retinoblastoma protein (pRb) induced by in vitro administration of Zebrafish embryonic extracts on human kidney adenocarcinoma cell line. *J. Tumor Marker Oncol.*, 2002, *17*(2), 59–64.

4. Cucina, A.; Biava, P.M.; D'Anselmi, F.; Coluccia, P.; Conti, F.; di Clemente, R.; Miccheli, A.; Frati, L.; Gulino, A.; Bizzarri, M. Zebrafish embryo proteins induce apoptosis in human colon cancer cells (Caco2). *Apoptosis*, 2006, *11*(9), 1617–1628.

5. Livraghi, T.; Meloni, F.; Frosi, A.; Lazzaroni, S.; Bizzarri, T. M.; Frati, L.; Biava, P.M. Treatment with stem cell differentiation stage factors of intermediate-advanced hepatocellular carcinoma: an open randomized clinical trial. *Oncol. Res.*, 2005, *15*(7–8), 399–408.

6. Livraghi, T. Ceriani, R. Palmisano, A. Pedicini, V. Pich, M. G. Tommasini, M.A. Torzilli, G. Complete response in 5 out of 38 patients with Advanced Hepatocellular Carcinoma treated with stem cell differentiation Stage Factors: Case Report from a single Center. *Curr. Pharm. Biotech.*, 2011, *12*(2).

7. Biava, P.M.; Canaider, S.; Facchin, F.; Bianconi, E.; Ljungberg, L.; Rotilio, D.; Burigana, F.; and Ventura, C. Stem Cell Differentiation Stage Factors from Zebrafish embryo: a novel strategy to modulate the fate of normal and pathological (stem) cells. *Curr. Pharm. Biotechnol.* 2015, *16*(9), 782–92.

8. Harak, H.; Frosi, A.; Biava, P.M. Studio clinico sull'efficacia e tollerabilita' di una crema per uso topico nel trattamento della psoriasi. *La Med. Biol.*, 2012, *3*, 27–31.

9. Calzavara-Pinton, P.; Rossi, M. A topical remedy in association with phototherapy. Efficacy evaluation in patients suffering from moderate psoriasis. *Hi.tech dermo*, 2012, *1*, 41–47.

10. Biava, P.M.; Bonsignorio, D. Cancer and cell differentiation: a model to explain malignancy. *J. Tumor Marker Oncol.*, 2002, *17*(2), 47–54.

11. Biava, P.M; Monguzzi, A; Bonsignorio, D; Frosi, A; Sell, S; Klavins J.V. Xenopus laevis Embryos share antigens with Zebrafish Embryos and with human malignant neoplasms. *J. Tumor Marker Oncol.*, 2001, *16*(3), 203–206.

12. Lawson, J.C.; Blatch, G.L.; Edkins, A.L. Cancer stem cells in breast cancer and metastasis. *Breast Cancer Res. Treat.*, 2009, *118*(2), 241–254.

13. Luo, J.; Yin, X.; Ma, T.; Lu, J. Stem cells in normal mammary gland and breast cancer. *Am. J. Med. Sci.*, 2010, *339*(4), 366–370.

14. Spiro, S. G.; Tanner, N. T.; Silvestri, G. A.; Janes, S. M.; Lim, E.; Vansteenkiste, J.F.; Pirker, R. Lung cancer: progress in diagnosis staging and therapy. *Respirology*, 2010, *15*(1), 44–50.

15. Gorelik, E.; Lokshin, A.; Levina, V. Lung cancer stem cells as a target for therapy. *Anticancer Agents Med. Chem.*, 2010, *10*(2), 164–171.

16. Sullivan, J.P.; Minna, J.D.; Shay, J.W. Evidence for self-renewing lung cancer stem cells and their implications in tumor initiation, progression and targeted therapy. *Cancer Metastasis Rev.*, 2010, *29*(1), 61–72.

17. Westhoff, B.; Colaluca, I.N.; D'Ario, G.; Donzelli, M.; Tosoni, D.; Volorio, S.; Pelosi, G.; Spaggiari, L.; Mazzarol, G.; Viale, G.; Pece, S.; Di Fiore,

P.P. Alterations of the Notch pathway in lung cancer. *Proc. Natl. Acad. Sci. USA*, 2009, *106*(52), 22293–22298.

18. Lang, S.H.; Anderson, E.; Fordham, R.; Collins, A.T. Modeling the prostate stem cell niche: an evaluation of stem cell survival and expansion in vitro. *Stem. Cells Dev.*, 2010, *19*(4), 537–546.

19. Joung, J.Y.; Cho, K.S.; Kim, J.E.; Seo, H.K.; Chung, J.; Park, W. S.; Choi, M.K.; Lee, K.H. Prostate stem cell antigen mRNA in peripheral blood as a potential predictor of biochemical recurrence of metastatic prostate cancer. *J. Surg. Oncol.*, 2010, *101*(2), 145–148.

20. Liu, T.; Cheng, W.; Lai, D.; Huang, Y.; Guo, L. Characterization of primary ovarian cancer cells in different culture systems. *Oncol. Rep.*, 2010, *23*(5), 1277–1284.

21. Fong, M.Y.; Kakar, S.S. The role of cancer stem cells and the side population in epithelial ovarian cancer. *Histol. Histopathol.*, 2010, *25*(1), 113–120.

22. Murphy, S.K. Targeting ovarian cancer-initiating cells. *Anticancer Agents Med. Chem.*, 2010, *10*(2), 157–163.

23. Peng, S.; Maihle, N.J.; Huang, Y. Pluripotency factors Lin 28 and Oct 4 identify a sub-population of stem cell-like cells in ovarian cancer. *Oncogene*, 2010, *29*(14), 2153–2159.

24. Tomuleasa, C.; Soritau, O.; Rus-Ciuca, D.; Pop, T.; Todea, D.; Mosteanu, O.; Pintea, B.; Foris, V.; Susman, S.; Kacso, G.; Irimie, A. Isolation and characterization of hepatic cells with stem-like properties from hepatocellular carcinoma. *J. Gastrointestin. Liver Dis.*, 2010, *19*(1), 61–67.

25. Zou, G.M. Liver cancer stem cells as an important target in liver cancer therapies. *Anticancer Agents Med. Chem.*, 2010, *10*(2), 172–175.

26. Lee, T.K.; Castilho, A.; Ma, S.; Ng, I.O. Liver cancer stem cells: implications for new therapeutic target. *Liver Int.,* 2009, *29*(7), 955–965.

27. Marquardt, J.U.; Thorgeirsson, S.S. Stem Cells in hepatocarcinogenesis: evidence from genomic data. *Semin. Liver Dis.*, 2010, *30*(1), 26–34.

28. Kung, J.W.; Currie, I.S.; Forbes, S.J.; Ross, J.A. Liver development, regeneration, and carcinogenesis. *J. Biomed. Biotechnol.*, 2010, *2010*, 984248.

29. Gai, H.; Nguyen, D.M.; Moon, Y.J.; Aguila, J.R.; Fink, L.M.; Ward, D.C.; Ma, Y. Generation of murine hepatic lineage cells from induced pluripotent stem cells. *Differentiation*, 2010, *79*(3), 171–181.

30. Correia, M.; Machado, J.C.; Ristimaki, A. Basic aspects of gastric cancer. *Helicobacter*, 2009, *14*(1), 36–40.

31. Takaishi, S.; Okumura,T.; Tu, S.; Wang, S.S.; Shibata, W.; Vigneshwaran, R.;

Gordon, S.A.; Shimada, Y.; Wang, T.C. Identification of gastric cancer stem cells using the surface marker CD44. *Stem Cells*, 2009, *27*(5), 1006–1020.

32. Nishii, T.; Yashiro, M.; Shinto, O.; Sawada, T.; Ohira, M.; Hirakawa, K. Cancer stem cell-like SP cells have a high adhesion ability to the peritoneum in gastric carcinoma. *Cancer Sci.*, 2009, *100*(8), 1397–1402.

33. Chen, Z.; Xu, W.R.; Qian, H.; Zhu, W.; Bu, X.F.; Wang, S.; Yan, Y.M.; Mao, F.; Gu, H.B.; Cao, H.L.; Xu, X.J. Oct4, a novel marker for human gastric cancer. *J. Surg. Oncol.*, 2009, *99*(7), 414–419.

34. Kang, D.H.; Han, M.E.; Song, M.H.; Lee, Y.S.; Kim, E.H.; Kim, H.J.; Kim, G.H.; Kim, D.H.; Yoon, S.; Baek, S.Y.; Kim, B.S.; Kim, J.B.; Oh, S.O. The role of hedgehog signaling during gastric regeneration. *J. Gastroenterol.*, 2009, *44*(5), 372–379.

35. Yeung, T.M.; Ghandhi, S.C.; Wilding, J.L.; Muschel, R.; Bodmer, W. F. Cancer stem cells from colorectal cancer derived cell lines. *Proc. Natl. Acad. Sci. USA*, 2010, *107*(8), 3722–3727.

36. Yeung, T.M.; Ghandhi, S.C.; Wilding, J.L.; Muschel, R.; Bodmer, W. F. Cancer stem cells from colorectal cancer derived cell lines. *Proc. Natl. Acad. Sci. USA*, 2010, *107*(8), 3722–3727.

37. Gulino, A.; Ferretti, E.; De Smaele, E. Hedgehog signaling in colon cancer and stem cells. *EMBO Mol. Med.*, 2009, *1*(6–7), 300–302.

38. Thenappan, A.; Li, Y.; Shetty, K.; Johnson, L.; Reddy, E.P.; Mishra, L. New therapeutic targeting colon cancer stem cells. *Curr. Colorectal Cancer Rep.*, 2009, *5*(4), 209.

39. Rasheed, Z.A.; Yang, J.; Wang, Q.; Kowalski, J.; Freed, I.; Murter, C.; Hong. S.M.; Koorstra, J. B.; Rajeshkumar, N.V.; He, X.; Goggins, M.; Iacobuzio-Donahue, C.; Berman, D.M.; Laheru, D.; Jimeno, A.; Hidalgo, M.; Maitra, A.; Matsui, W. Prognostic significance of tumorigenic cells with mesenchymal features in pancreatic adenocarcinoma. *J. Natl. Cancer Inst.*, 2010, *102*(5), 340–351.

40. Puri, S.; Hebrok, M. Cellular plasticity within pancreas-lessons learned from development. *Dev. Cell*, 2010, *18*(3), 342–356.

41. Quante, M.; Wang,T. C. Stem cells in gastroenterology and hepatology. *Nat. Rev. Gastroenterol. Hepatol.*, 2009, *6*(12), 724–737.

42. Ailles, L.; Prince, M. Cancer stem cells in head and neck squamous cell carcinoma. *Methods Mol. Biol.*, 2009, *568*, 175–193.

43. Zhang, P.; Zhang, Y.; Mao, L.; Zhang, Z.; Chen, W. Side population in oral squamous cell carcinoma possesses tumor stem cell phenotype. *Cancer Lett.*, 2009, *277*(2), 227–234.

44. Brunner M.; Thurnher, D.; Heiduschka, G.; Grasl, M.Ch.; Brostjan, C.; Erovic, B.M. Elevated levels of circulating endothelial progenitor cells in head and neck cancer patients. *J. Surg. Oncol.*, 2008, *98*(7), 545–550.

45. Zhang, Q.; Shi, S.; Yen, Y.; Brown, J.; Ta, J. Q.; Le, A. D. A subpopulation of CD133(+) cancer stem-like cells characterized in human oral squamous cell carcinoma confer resistance to chemotherapy. *Cancer Lett.*, 2010, *289*(2), 151–160.

46. Sato, A.; Sakurada, K.; Kumabe, T.; Sasajima, T.; Beppu, T.; Asano, K.; Ohkuma, H.; Ogawa, A.; Mizoi, K.; Tominaga, T.; Kitanaka, C.; Kayama, T.; Tohoku Brain Tumor Study Group. Association of stem cell marker CD133 expression with dissemination of glioblastoma. *Neurosurg. Rev.*, 2010, *33*(2), 175–183.

47. Di Tomaso, T.; Mazzoleni, S.; Wang, E.; Sovena, G.; Clavenna, D.; Franzin, A.; Mortini, P.; Ferrone, S.; Doglioni, C.; Marincola, F. M.; Galli, R.; Parmiani, G.; Maccalli, C. Immunobiological characterization of cancer stem cells isolated from glioblastoma patients. *Clin. Cancer Res.*, 2010, *16*(3), 800–813.

48. Ji, J.; Black, K.L.; Yu, J.S. Glioma stem cell research for the development of immunotherapy. *Neurosurg. Clin. N. Am.*, 2010, *21*(1), 159–166.

49. Biava, P. M.; Fiorito, A.; Negro, C.; Mariani, M. Effects of treatment with embryonic and uterine tissue homogenates on Lewis lung carcinoma development. *Cancer Letters,* 1988, *41*(3); 265–70.

50. Biava, P.M.; Carluccio, A. Activation of anti-oncogene p53 produced by embryonic extracts in vitro tumor cells. *J. Tumor Marker Oncol.*, 1977, *12*(4), 9–15.

51. Biava, P.M.; Bonsignorio, D.; Hoxa, M.; Facco, R.; Ielapi, T.; Frati, L.; Bizzarri, M. "Post-translational modification of the retinoblastoma protein (pRb) induced by in vitro administration of Zebrafish embryonic extracts on human kidney adenocarcinoma cell line.: *J. Tumor Marker Oncology,* 2002, *17*(2); 59–64.)

52. Biava, P.M.; Bonsignorio, D.; Hoxa, M. Cell proliferation curves of different human tumor lines after in vitro treatment with Zebrafish embryonic extracts. *J. Tumor Marker Oncol.*, 2001, *16*(3), 195–202.

53. Biava, P.M.; Bonsignorio, D.; Hoxha, M.; Impagliazzo, M.; Frosi, A.; Larese, F.; Negro, C. Mother-embryo cross-talk: the anti-cancer substances produced by mother and embryo during cell differentiation. A review of experimental data. *J. Tumor Marker Oncol.*, 2002, *17,* 55–58.

54. Livraghi, T.; Meloni, F.; Frosi, A.; Lazzaroni, S.; Bizzarri, M; Frati, L.; Biava, P.M. Treatment with stem cell differentiation stage factors of intermediate-advanced hepatocellular carcinoma: an open randomized clinical trial. *Oncol. Res.,* 2005, *15,* 399–408.

CHAPTER III

Summing Up:
The Meaning of Information
Medicine for Our Life
and Times

The paradigm discussed in this study is a radical innovation in the context of conventional wisdom, but its insights are not new; they have been known for millennia. The universe is not a material system, but a cosmic information network. It "runs" on information. The information—more precisely the "in-formation"—on which it runs is the basis of persistence in that network, and sustained contact and communication with it is the secret of flourishing in the network.

This insight has been stated in the wisdom traditions in the language of their place and time. It is restated and reaffirmed in the language and cognitive framework of contemporary science. *The universe is a "macroscopic quantum system of in-formed vibration," and the organism is an intrinsic segment of that in-formation. The cosmic information that "forms" the universe also forms—"in-forms"—the organism.*

Alignment with the in-formation that structures and forms the organism is the key to maintaining its health. The level of alignment with this "in-formation" decides whether an organism is healthy and flourishing, merely vegetating at the margins of survival, or is moribund in the grips of disease.

We are in constant contact with the in-formation that acts on our organism, but the level of our contact can vary. It can be weak and may also be largely suppressed. Then, like a recessive gene, although the in-formation needed for our health and well-being is given, it is not active. When contact and communication are repressed, the vitality of the organism is impaired, and the very survival of the organism is in question.

The revolutionary discovery reported here is a clear and convincing example of the application of science's new paradigm to a wide range of interest. The insights and principles of the new paradigm in medicine are not just theoretical abstractions. They are functional mappings of real-world processes. The range of their application encompasses fields as diverse as physics and cosmology, the cognitive and the social sciences—and the sciences of life, including the science of medicine.*

In information medicine, science's new paradigm finds highly focused application. The universal governing and structuring attractor present in nature is the highest-level factor active in the explicate order. Information medicine seeks contact with this factor and achieves it inter alia through extracts from a living embryo. These extracts are stem cell differentiating factors, and they are able to reprogram mutant and malignant stem cells to normalcy.

This is an epochal discovery. The exploration of its implications and applications can fundamentally change the face of modern medicine. The following seven assessments speak to this point from a variety of perspectives of actual and potential interest.

---

*A more complete listing and description of the range of application of the new paradigm is provided in Ervin Laszlo, *The Handbook of New Paradigm Research,* 2018 (ISBN-13: 978-1-945390-25-8 print edition; ISBN-13: 978-1-945390-26-5 e-book edition).

SEVEN ASSESSMENTS

Raoul Goldberg

PATH to Health Integrative Medical Centre, Cape Town, S.A.

As a wide-eyed, curious medical student, I watched chick embryos grow and develop in so precise and perfect a manner, that I knew then there had to be some invisible guiding in-forming principle directing this living maturation process. Later the study of human embryology took me on a miraculous flow experience of life unfolding in simultaneous synchronous patterns of such exquisite precision and beauty that the in-streaming river of in-formation was palpably present. Ervin Laszlo and Pier Mario Biava, with their seminal book on the in-formation paradigm and its application to medical research, direct our awareness to these highly evolved in-forming forces in the universe that carry the ordered patterns of all forms within their force fields—forces that manifest materially and holographically in all the shapes and forms of the seemingly material world right down to the finest matter-like particles.

Rudolf Steiner named these universal forces *etheric formative forces,* whose four main etheric force fields—warmth, light, sound-chemical, and life forces—are the procreators of all forms and substances through their intercreative and interweaving dynamic activities. Each has specific form-giving characteristics: warmth etheric is generative-forming, light etheric is form and shape-differentiating, sound-chemical etheric is member-differentiating, and life etheric is life- and wholeness-forming. Thus the force that generates the unfoldment of the seed is the warmth etheric force; the light etheric will then determine the overall form—for example, too much light will restrict the size of the leaf but will create a more differentiated form (e.g., fern compared to water pond leaves); the sound formative force will create the different organs or members of an organism; and the life etheric force will give form to the various life processes that together hold the organism in a formed wholeness. All processes and substances in the world are shaped by these form-giving forces, from the galaxial nebulae to the heart or larynx; to the animals, plants, fish, insects, shells, crystals; to the embryonic forms; and to molecular and atomic formations. In the language of David Bohm, the *implicate order* harbors these innate formative forces, unfolding the *explicate manifest order* of the sense-perceptible world.

The common features and differences of embryonic stem cells and cancer cells are well established, but what is exceptional and exciting about this book is on the one hand the recognition of the in-forming and form-giving forces that impart correct information for healthy cell growth and differentiation, and on the other hand the use of embryonic stem cells in the re-in-forming shaping therapy of cancer cells. Healthy stem cells are an *explicit manifestation of the implicit field of in-formation.* Cancer cells have lost their connection to this in-streaming intelligence, and the self-regulating forces of the body and mind are not able to control this dis-ordered and dis-informed cell life. The sum total of epigenetic external and internal environmental pressures that trigger genetic misinformation is the underlying dynamic that leads to this disruption. Principally it is the human mind that makes unhealthy life choices and sets down dysfunctional habitual patterns, leading to a chronic stress syndrome that disconnects the human being from nature's ordered stream of in-formation.

This book gifts us in extraordinary ways: it informs us and reconnects us to that pristine in-forming field of reality that underlies our existence. Our activity of thinking, as Steiner describes, comes from this same sphere of in-formation and is the refined force of biological growth and form. By aligning ourselves with these form-giving forces, we can reconnect to the ordered stream of life. Furthermore, it opens up a field of medical research that has the potential to reorder the entire biological domain, to counteract disease predispositions, reverse disease conditions, and invigorate health.

Maria Sagi

The Club of Budapest

For more than twenty years, in addition to working for the Club of Budapest, I have been researching, writing, and practicing an information-based form of natural healing. During this time I could confirm time and time again that the right kind of information, applied with the right method by a qualified physician or healer, can literally work wonders. Let me briefly clarify and substantiate this claim.

The information addressed in "in-formation medicine" is not the human-created information we know in our daily life. It is the deep information—the "in-formation" that, according to David Bohm, forms and permeates the manifest universe. Healing with in-formation is not a supernatural or extrascientific undertaking. It is to make practical use of the in-formation—a cosmic attractor—that structures events in space and time. The attractor that forms and in-forms events in space and time forms and in-forms the living organism. This "in-formation" can be facilitated and reinforced. Doing so is the task of the in-formation medicine presented in this book.

The cosmic attractor that forms and in-forms systems in the universe acts through the quantum field, which is the underlying reality of the universe. In terms of the new physics discussed by Laszlo and Biava, that field is a space-time domain of coherent vibration. The patterns that appear in that domain "in-form" systems in the manifest universe. They in-form living systems, including human beings. These are complex and coherent systems, but the level of their coherence is various, and it can change over time. In the human world, a significant reduction in the level of coherence of a system indicates a condition of ill health, and possibly the presence of disease.

The coherence of the human organism can be raised, and ultimately reestablished at the healthy level, by introducing the in-formation that acts on the system. Access to that in-formation can reprogram faulty cellular and multicellular processes, as convincingly demonstrated by the pioneering research of Pier Mario Biava.

In my own work, the key to healing with in-formation is to match two kinds of patterns in the embedding quantum field. That field, called by Laszlo "Akashic Field," is a universal memory field and everything that happens in space and time leaves its mark in it. These marks form recognizable patterns of vibration. Some patterns mark particular, quasi-individual (but not radically separate) events, and others mark entire classes and ensembles of events.

There are patterns that correspond to our individual organism: these are what I have called morphogenetic patterns. More general patterns code the class or species to which an organism belongs: these I call species-specific patterns. Evidently, there are still more general patterns; those, for example, that code the entire class of complex and coherent systems, including the subclass of living systems.

My concern as a natural healer is with the relation between the individual's own morphogenetic pattern and his or her species-specific pattern. The latter codes the norms of healthy functioning in human beings. I have come to realize that relating the individual's particular morphogenetic pattern to the general pattern of the species can heal malfunctions in the body: it introduces the attractor that can reprogram cells and cellular systems for normalcy. The manifest effect is the maximization of the flow of energy in the body. But for this to occur, the in-formation received by the individual organism must be brought into alignment with the in-formation that constitutes normal functioning in the body. This calls for the insertion of a pattern—a code of organic functioning—that the organism can receive and by which it can be "in-formed." Biava's discovery shows that this code is present in a wide variety of living systems, even in fish, and can heal mutant and imperfectly differentiated stem cells in the organism into which it is inserted.

The nature of the malfunction is a critical factor in healing with in-formation. Does the malfunction concern only the functionality of the organism, or is it of such magnitude that it impairs and modifies entire organs and organ systems? The in-formation medicine discovered by Biava can reprogram even radically impaired organs, such as those impaired by malignant tumors. In my vocabulary, healing cancer calls for reprogramming imperfectly differentiated or malignant cells by exposure to the in-formation coded by humanity's species-specific pattern. Access to that pattern can be attained by different means—in Biava's discovery it is attained by introducing a complex set of proteins extracted at particular points in the interaction of a Zebrafish with its embryo.

Biava's discovery is a towering achievement of modern medicine: it applies the in-formation that was hitherto missing in the treatment of chronic diseases. This in-formation, analogously to the activation of self-healing processes in the organism by ancient techniques, heals the organism without recourse to biochemical, biophysical, or surgical interventions, and without damaging side effects. It is cost-effective and does not damage the environment.

The healing I have been practicing for two decades has the same objective as that of Biava, but it uses a different method for attaining it. It is based on the discovery of the Austrian scientist Erich Körbler of a vector system that permits a reliable form of diagnosis. My development of the Körbler method permits me to diagnose the match or mismatch between the individual's morphogenetic pattern and the human species-specific pattern, and this in turn enables me to identify the substance that carries the information that can reinforce the match and can thus heal the malfunction. This method has proven its effectiveness in a wide variety of cases.

Healing with in-formation is an old and now rediscovered form of healing. Its power and range of application are not yet fully explored. But we have already good reason to believe that, as Biava and Laszlo maintain, its advent marks a new era in the history of medicine.

Dwight McKee

Integrative Cancer Consulting, Aptos, CA

Biava and Laszlo have written a most interesting, important, and I would go so far as to say *seminal* book about cancer, neuroprotection, aging, consciousness, and indeed, the very nature of reality. Although ostensibly about Dr. Biava's work with stem cell differentiation factors derived from Zebrafish embryos, the implications, both scientific and philosophical, go far beyond cancer, which has been the focus of my own work for over forty years.

A long time ago I realized that we can learn far more and advance much more rapidly if we view cancer as a teacher, a puzzle to be studied, rather than as an enemy to be vanquished (which all too often has resulted in the vanquishing of the patient in the process). As Dr. Biava points out in the discussion of his own decades of research, and what this book confirms, is that what cancer requires is "in-formation"—and until it receives it, it will continue to behave in a malignant way.

About twenty years ago I realized that the medical science of oncology is totally focused on ways to destroy tumor cells. Absolutely no attention has been paid to the environment of those tumor cells—to what I like to refer to as the internal "terrain" of the person who has cancer. Our internal terrain, which we now know to be shaped minute by minute, indeed second by second, even nanosecond by nanosecond by the process termed "epigenetics," is discussed in detail in this book. Everything we eat, drink, breathe, eliminate, think, feel, and use our bodies for contributes to this continuous dance that determines which genes are expressed, and which are not. It is this process that has led us to the understanding that our health and well-being is determined about 20 percent by the genes we inherit from our parents, and 80 percent by our nutrition, lifestyle, environment, relationships, thoughts, feelings, intentions, and beliefs—the factors that in combination influence the dynamic flow of the epigenetic process. At last, cancer research is beginning to focus on the so-called "tumor microenvironment" (TME), the makeup of which is equally determined by the activity of the tumor and the activity of the host. Tumor behavior can be dramatically influenced by nutrition, exercise, stress, fear, confidence, anger, hate, and love, simply by altering the environment in which the tumors grow—the environment that has been dubbed the TME.

I was impressed and excited when I first read the work of Dr. Beatrice Mintz, who in the mid-1970s did the first experiment that I am aware of using a highly lethal strain of cancer cells (teratocarcinoma), which, if injected into an adult mouse, predictably caused lethal tumors. The same strain, when injected into mouse embryos, turned out to have no effect on embryonic development. The resulting healthy newborn mice expressed all the genes of the otherwise lethal teratocarcinoma, but they were expressed in a healthy way. Very few people understood the implications of this experiment at the time, but Dr. Biava did and carried it even further. He discovered that the proteins expressed during the development of the Zebrafish embryo are essentially the same as those of any other embryo, and that when cancer cells are exposed to this "in-formation" they can become normal healthy cells, much as cancer cells do when injected into a mouse embryo during the period of organogenesis (when the organs are forming).

Dr. Mina Bissell did similar work in the 1980s with the Rous sarcoma virus, which causes deadly sarcoma tumors in chickens and other birds. She found that it would only produce a tumor when exposed to the terrain that we call a wound. If injected into a chicken, the tumor would occur only at the site of the wound (the injection site). And as Mintz had done a decade earlier, Bissell found that injecting the tumor-forming virus into early-stage chicken embryos does not produce tumors. So it seems the context—the environment, the terrain—in which a tumor cell finds itself is a powerful determinant of whether that cell continues to behave malignantly or differentiates into a normal healthy stem cell. The potential for differentiation into normal functionality is always present. We just have to find a way to shape the organism's internal environment and provide the proper systems of information for it. This is what the "in-formation" medicine described in this book vitally contributes to.

Dr. Biava's many decades of research with Zebrafish embryo stem cell differentiation stage factors (SCDSFs) has shown that they are also capable of profound neuroprotection against various toxic insults to nerve cells and can also slow the aging process of cells in general. As Laszlo and Biava so elegantly state in this book, these systems of information provided by SCDSFs are like an orchestra that can interpret many different symphonies.

I see this work as the dawn of a completely new and exciting era in medicine—one that has the potential to transform the way we diagnose, treat, and even think about the many malfunctions of living organisms we call "disease." Restoring complete in-formation to a dysfunctional living organism literally recreates "ease" from "disease."

I invite readers to go on a mind-bending ride with Laszlo and Biava—they may never again think about cancer and other diseases in the same way. And they will turn to the in-formation present in potential in all things, which may be the best medicine of all for organic diseases.

Larry Dossey

Explore: The Journal of Science and Healing

There are moments in the history of science that profoundly redirect the practice of medicine. Legendary examples include physician William Harvey's (1578–1657) description of the body's circulation; when Anton van Leeuwenhoek (1632–1723), a Dutch drapery merchant, peered down a simple microscope and described for the first time single-cell organisms he called animalcules, which we now call microorganisms; and when the Hungarian physician Ignaz Semmelweis (1818–1865) discovered that the incidence of lethal puerperal or childbed fever could be drastically reduced if obstetricians simply washed their hands with a chlorinated lime solution. It may be that the research findings of Pier Mario Biava encountered in this book will rank as an equally memorable moment.

This extraordinary research reveals a way of reversing serious illnesses that departs from conventional approaches. These experiments with cancer and other diseases have been conducted across two decades. They have been published in respected peer-reviewed journals. They involve, most notably, liver cancer (hepatocellular carcinoma or HCC) in intermediate and advanced stages following treatment by the administration of stem cell differentiation stage factors (SCDSFs). These are substances extracted from Zebrafish embryos during the stem cell differentiating process. Stem cell differentiation stage factors regulate the expression of genes; that is, the epigenetic code. As Dr. Biava elaborates, "[T]he molecular mechanisms at the basis of the slowdown of tumor growth due to treatment with SCDSF can be summed up as follows: cessation of the cell cycle in accordance with the type of tumor, genetic damage repair, and cell re-differentiation—or the apoptosis (death) of the tumor cells (if repair is no longer possible)."

The prognosis of liver cancer is abysmal. The American Cancer Society states the overall five-year survival rate for all stages of liver cancer is 15 percent. Many factors are at play. If the liver cancer is localized, confined to the liver, the five-year survival rate is 28 percent. If the liver cancer is regional, having grown into nearby organs, the five-year survival rate is 7 percent. Once the liver cancer has spread to distant organs or tissues, the survival time is as low as two years. Survival rates can be extended by available treatments. Liver cancers that can be surgically removed have a five-year survival rate of over 50 percent When detected in the earliest stages and a donor liver is transplanted, the five-year survival rate can be as high as 70 percent.[1]

How does therapy with SCDSFs compare? Dr. Biava states, "Results show that 19.8 percent of the patients experienced a regression and 16 percent of the patients experienced stabilization with an overall survival after 40 months of more than 60 percent of the patients who responded, compared with 10 percent of the non-responding patients. A wide improvement of performance status has been registered in a great majority of patients (82.6 percent), including in those who are in the progressive phase of the disease. A recent study of reprogramming normal and cancerous stem cells confirms the role of SCDSFs in producing a complete response in 13.1 percent patients experiencing primitive, intermediate, or advanced liver cancer."

Primary liver cancer is a major health problem globally. It is the sixth most frequent cancer and is the second leading cause of death from cancer worldwide.[2] In 2012 it occurred in 782,000 people and in 2015 resulted in 810,500 deaths.[3,4] In 2015, 263,000 deaths from liver cancer were due to hepatitis B, 167,000 to hepatitis C, and 245,000 to alcohol. Higher rates of liver cancer occur where hepatitis B and C are common, including Asia and sub-Saharan Africa.[5] Males are more often affected with HCC than females. Diagnosis is most frequent among those fifty-five to sixty-five years old. In the United States, five-year survival rates overall are 18 percent.[6]

Therapeutic options include surgery, liver transplantation, ablation (killing cancer cells using heat, laser, or injecting special compounds directly into the cancer), embolization of particles or beads to block the blood supply to the cancer, radiation, or chemotherapy. All current therapies are associated with side effects ranging from mild to severe.

The contrast between the mode of action of conventional therapies and Biava's SCDSFs is striking. SCDSFs operate in an "informational" sense, reprogramming aberrant cell function and directing it back on track.

We have become used to cancer treatments that are invasive, destructive, and fraught with unpleasant side effects. The possibility of another approach—informational reinstruction or redirection of biological processes gone awry—seems almost fictional. Yet that is the option presented by Dr. Biava's research. He offers what can be considered an "upstream" approach compared with the "downstream" approach of conventional therapies.

Here we encounter philosophical issues. Philosophies of medicine and science are often excoriated by professionals as worthless obstructions to practicality and getting things done. As the Nobel Prize–winning physicist Richard Feynman once said, "Philosophy of science is about as useful to scientists as ornithology is to birds."[7] And as the maxim often quoted by surgeons states, "To cut is to cure." In other words, get on with things; don't fool around with time-wasting, airy-fairy philosophizing.

Yet we must be mindful of the philosophical underpinnings of what we do in medicine, or we will drift into automatized thinking and doing. As evidence of this drift, consider the *Merck Manual,* a massive tome published periodically in the United States as a reference guide to the thousands of pharmaceuticals available to physicians. The nineteenth edition, published in 2011, contains nearly four thousand pages, prompting some physicians to describe it in terms of pounds instead of page count. The index includes sixty categories of "anti" pharmaceuticals, each category representing many items. The categories range alphabetically from antiandrogens to antivirals. Around half the four thousand pages are devoted to side effects. That said, these medications are mainstays of our allopathic approach, and collectively they have saved countless lives, as in the case of antibiotics, for which we should be deeply grateful. Yet whether one approves of medical philosophy or not, these sixty categories embody a particular philosophy—an oppositional or combative approach to health problems, obvious in the "anti" prefix in the name of all sixty categories that include hundreds of medications.

The SCDSF-based approach invokes a different strategy. These compounds reorient aberrant biological pathways at critical points in cellular maturation and development. This is not a "better" approach in a moral sense, but it definitely appears superior in terms of fewer side effects and less suffering that patients experience during treatments. This situation is analogous to the contrast between prevention and medical-surgical intervention. Prevention is not dramatic; it can be so simple and down-to-earth that it appears trivial; yet the unglamorous "upstream" approach of prevention is to be favored wherever evidence supports its effectiveness.

Here is an inescapable fact: in science and medicine we are haunted by philosophy. The attempt to avoid its influence is a fool's errand. We may ignore its impact in the therapies we elect and the experiments we pursue, but philosophical vectors are always present. They usually operate unconsciously. Consider the following passage by historian of science Carolyn Merchant in her discussion of Sir Francis Bacon's role in the early days of science, before "science" was even an accepted term:

Nature for Francis Bacon and nearly everyone else in the Renaissance and Scientific Revolution was female. More than a metaphor, Nature was the servant of God in the mundane world—the bringer and reproducer of life and the meter of rewards and punishments. Accepted as both reality and metaphor by the lower, as well as the upper classes, Nature represented a fusion of ancient, Renaissance, and Christian symbols. Depicted as female by a host of artists, writers, philosophers, and ordinary people, Nature was a personification of the cosmos, the earth, and the human writ large. . . . All aspects of the body were symbolized by the female, the weaker and more vulnerable sex. Matter, too, as female, represented the lower order of nature. Matter, like the female, was inconstant, changing, and corruptible. Matter, the body, and the reproductive organs were sites of potential corruption by the devil. *To deny this reality of daily moral life is to discount history itself* [emphasis added].[8]

Our metaphors give us away. Consider how we have long spoken of the heart as a "pump" and its components as "valves," a hydrological salute to the influence of the Industrial Revolution; how we refer to the liver as a "filter;" or how we've upgraded to present-day terms in describing the brain as a "supercomputer" and DNA as a "code." This is not all bad. Because metaphors help us express how we function, they are an unavoidable linguistic tool and a wonderful one if used wisely.

Liver cancer is not the only disease that responds to SCDSF therapy. This book also reports on experiments regarding other functions of the epigenetic code, functions that can not only reprogram tumor cells, but can also prevent neurodegenerative processes, significantly ameliorate psoriasis, stop processes of senescence, and increase the life span of cells. So although we do not know the limits of these therapies, it is likely they extend beyond specific diseases, perhaps to the aging process itself. For as Biava says: "The results of anti-aging treatments and the prevention of neurodegenerative disorders point to the same processes: the differentiation factors are epigenetic regulators with different specific functions. They are like an orchestra that can interpret different symphonies. . . . Life is organized on the basis of information programs that provide integral and precise instruction packages: these packages act as integral wholes. If they are fragmented, they lose their effectiveness."

In this book Biava and Laszlo emphasize the fundamental uniqueness of these findings. Their research introduces a new phase in the evolution of medicine. It shifts the center of attention from a mechanistic to a systemic concept, to the realization that the system of life is essentially an information network.

Biava's and Laszlo's approach to "in-formation" reminds me of anthropologist and social scientist Gregory Bateson's definition of information: it is a difference that makes a difference. This is a major shift in medical thought, as different from conventional medical thinking as quantum-relativistic concepts in physics differ from mechanical, classical, Newtonian principles. In observing Biava's work, it is as if we are witnessing something as significant as van Leeuwenhoek's seeing his animalcules for the first time.

If, as seems likely, this research significantly relieves human suffering worldwide, Pier Mario Biava will come to stand in medicine's pantheon alongside giants such as van Leeuwenhoek, Harvey, Semmelweis, and many other visionaries whose insights have diminished human misery and increased the probability that the human spirit will soar.

Giulio Sapelli

University of Milan

The reflections on the outcome of the globalization and the capitalism that dominates our planet continue with questionable scientific results, but with strong effect on public common sense. The book by Laszlo and Biava is a decisive contribution to defeating the diseases of our time by creating a robust scientific basis that goes beyond current common sense in building a new paradigm for thought and action. The value of their contribution is due to its deeply interdisciplinary nature, moving beyond the absolutist and exclusivist thought that has prevailed for the past thirty years and prevented the sound understanding of society and of social relations. It stood in the way of finding the way that has become necessary to overcome the world's problems.

Today's absolutist and exclusivist thought produced an analytical individualist-behaviorist perspective and a materialistic and acquisitive anthropological hypothesis: the unlimited rationality of individuals bent on maximizing their pecuniary utilities. The thought of the authors of this important work is the opposite of the popular, crude materialistic hypothesis that derives culturally from the neoclassical position in economics and the neoliberal ideology in politics.

In context of the epistemologically holistic hypothesis put forward in this book, the current perception of globalization as a mainly economic and basically new phenomenon emerges from the uninterrupted advance of modernity, even though it is already transcended in the advent of postmodern capitalism. The thought of Laszlo and Biava shuns common sense and lays the foundations for research that goes beyond public prejudices and the analytical reduction of complexity. It refuses common sense clichés and puts the world back on its feet—to cite the metaphor of a master of an already nearly forgotten system of thought.

The contemporary world is turned on its head by the exclusion of the science of life, of the living human being, and of the knowledge essential for those who are responsible for the management of the diverse strata of society.

Today's transformation is not a linear, faint, and mechanical process. Those who are responsible for managing the diverse strata of society believe that they have succeeded in their aims and shout victory, yet they are only following a path dictated by chance. Their victory comes by distorting events in an illusory narrative that does not reflect conditions in reality. Their processes of communication change perceptions and dispense fables instead of realistic narratives. In this way, the possibilities of finding a cure to our problems are blocked. History and care for life as a concrete phenomenon cannot be reduced to graphs that measure (or are believed to measure) changing appearances and ignore the causes. They transmute the transformation with a succession of icons, instead of depicting it realistically as Renaissance paintings can do.

The cure, according to the authors, proves to be a practical application of moral philosophy, based on an anthropologically sound image of humans. This is the case even if the medical professional in today's world—a world that is getting more and more fragmented and self-referential—remains unaware of it in the context of the stupefying ignorance of mainstream society.

For the dominant ideology, the image that prevails is that of the individual as a liberal mathematically formulated archetype. But for the revolutionaries who embrace the perspective offered in this book, the image is the nonquantifiable, irreducible, and irreproducible person at the center of every attempt at caring and healing.

In the dominant view, the marketplace of human well-being is probabilistic, only "nearly perfect," but in fact dominated by rampant imperfection and subject to the cyclic nature of socioeconomic growth as well as of depression and crisis. The new approach interprets the current zeitgeist as arising from the rubble of crisis. The truth of this is shown by the resistance that people manifest in the face of crisis, evidencing strong and often unexpected resilience, joining and uniting more than it appears on first sight. The current transformation makes evident networks that emerge from the crisis itself—cooperative cultures that in the mainstream perspective are not even admitted and, when visible, are not seen. . . .

The polyarchic undemocratic face of the world capitalist order, with its exclusivist thought and single market dominance, is no longer private. It is as public as the European polyarchies are that pretend to be technocracies. Imposing its consequences on the market created the decadence in which we are immersed today. This form of society can no longer create meaning and therefore lacks vital motivation. Meaning has become divorced from function.

The market governs itself and proceeds toward the ruin of the weakest and the victory of the ruling polyarchies. Profit becomes the dizzying illusion of the power to control risk; it is a weapon of mass destruction, blind in the face of the relative poverty that spreads and cannot be exorcised. Absolute poverty stands in the way of any transformation that could prevent the oncoming of a collapse.

Change or fall into the abyss: that is the alternative that confronts the world at the beginning of the third decade of this millennium. There is no escape. The unstable technocracy proclaimed by business schools has failed. It collapsed, and the plebiscitary democracy, which is about to become the most relevant political mechanism for creating a society of rights, is likewise failing.

When trust in uninterrupted consumption collapses, plebiscitary democracy, not backed by a strong state of law and order, reveals itself as an instrument of homologization, in the service of an equality à la Tocqueville. But even this possibility has been destroyed by the market: only the right of the merchants remains. This, however, is insufficient to govern society, even when supported by the moral suasion of the rulers of the international market.

Placing money, rather than work, as the pillar of social organization has had devastating consequences. Money is not capable of restructuring classes, roles, social functions, and is not able to reaggregate the social system and make it into a meaningful, productive community.

This step created the disastrous condition in which we are immersed today. Without any other legitimacy than that of money controlled by the great bankers, recent events in the world are indications of a general transformation.

The book of Laszlo and Biava, in stark contract with the dominant ideology, suggests an exit from the crisis produced by the reactivation of a nonstatist neocommunal model. In addition to offering a revolutionary new scientific perspective, Laszlo and Biava put forward a courageous moral perspective. They propose a change of paradigm that goes beyond the field of medicine and challenges us to commit ourselves to the construction of a new world.

Kingsley Dennis
The Laszlo Institute of New Paradigm Research

We are in a privileged position in being witnesses to the birthing—and breakthrough—of new paradigm perspectives into the world. We are truly on the cusp of revolutionary discoveries in all areas of human understanding. As Thomas Kuhn indicated in his *The Structure of Scientific Revolutions* over half a century ago, such dramatic leaps occur when enough new evidence (or, as he termed them, "anomalies") start to encroach on the incumbent mainstream narrative. It has been our intention at the Laszlo Institute of New Paradigm Research to work toward gathering new-paradigm investigations in areas such as science, health, business, consciousness studies, politics, the economy, and more. Within all disciplines and in all areas, this indicates that the new paradigm is no longer either wishful thinking or a peripheral perspective. It is the upcoming perception of how life, the universe, and all things work and need to be considered.

Laszlo and Biava are riding this revolutionary cusp with their seminal research into the fundamental nature of medicine and its implications for the conquest of disease and the extension of the span of human life. The foundations for this understanding were laid out in one of the author's previous works. In the books *What Is Reality?* and *The Intelligence of the Cosmos*, Ervin Laszlo posited an understanding that the universe (our space-time matrix) is not made up from bits of matter but from clusters of highly ordered "in-formed" energy-vibration. Furthermore, the primary driver of evolution in the universe—the basic "attractor"—is toward coherence. As Laszlo has pointed out, the universe is a coherent system of interacting and coevolving clusters of vibration. The new paradigm in science tells us that the universe is not a mechanical system but, on the contrary, operates akin to a "cosmic information-network." The universe is universally in-formed: it literally "runs" on information.

For the purposes of this book, Laszlo and Biava have taken this fundamental insight and applied it to modern medicine. Just as coherence is the evolutionary attractor in the universe, so it is that for the sustained health of the living organism. Alignment is the key to health and wellbeing in the domains of life; and this alignment corresponds to coherent contact with nature's in-formation. As the authors show, contact and communication with this in-formation can be "effectively oriented" and "purposively enhanced." Illness is the manifestation of blockages of in-formation, and the task of medicine is to investigate ways and means to overcome them. New-paradigm medicine is about maintaining and strengthening overall harmony and balance with the in-formation that shapes and structures the world.

New-paradigm medicine is not just a theoretical postulate. Laszlo and Biava show with strong scientifically accredited research that it works in clinical practice. Dr. Biava's research on stem cell differentiation factors derived from Zebrafish embryos has provided astounding results in the treatment of cancer patients. While the research in this book largely focuses on the reprogramming of cancer stem-like cells, the implications, both scientific and philosophical, go far beyond cancer. New-paradigm medicine shifts the foundation of the medical enterprise from a mechanistic to a systemic concept.

In order to understand the framework of new-paradigm medicine, we need to shift our view of how we perceive the structure of reality. The publication of this seminal book constitutes a turning point not only in medicine and in science, but in our most fundamental conception of life and the universe—of the real world.

Alessandro Pizzoccaro

Guna Terapia d'avanguardia, Milan

It is a great honor for me to comment on the latest book written by two scientists for whom I have enormous admiration. My admiration has increased after reading this work, one that offers a paramount and sound vision and explanation of nothing less than the Universe, Evolution and Medicine in a unified concept.

This unified interpretation is so important today, when specialization in science, technology, and social and humanistic studies dominates the concept of knowledge and of life. Thus there is a serious risk that society assumes senseless directions, lacking a guiding star. This is a risk for the future of humanity itself.

The unified vision of the macro and the micro dimensions of the universe offered in this book, together with the related coherent interpretation of health and sickness, helps to give sense to human existence and offers a logical understanding of everyday life.

Many of the concepts discussed in this book have been part of the patrimony of the community of science, but the value of the book is the integration of the most important of these theories and discoveries in an integral vision. To mention only the most important discoveries, I shall cite the recognition that space is not empty, but on the contrary full of energies manifested by frequencies and vibrations—a concept that was put forward by Nikola Tesla already a century ago. As a result, the reality we perceive through our senses is illusory. The perceived material world is merely the representation we give to the range of the frequencies perceivable by us. The deepest reality is an infinite sequence of frequencies, amazingly coherent and cooperative. If it were not for this condition, the whole universe would collapse in global chaos. This enormously finely tuned universe has been existing for billions of years following the Big Bang and may continue to exist for additional billions of years.

We still face great and complex mysteries, but it is now clear at least that the matrix of the universe is "in-formation," a system that is structured and coherent, all-inclusive, holistically integrated, and in continuous evolution . . . toward what ultimate end, nobody knows. This is a mystery that not even the new paradigm discussed in this book can explain. But it is certain that the new paradigm reinforces the need to recognize an immanent or transcendent Creator. The vision of Laszlo and Biava excludes the possibility that the universe, and the life generated in it, is the product of mere fortuitous coincidences.

The interpretation in this book of the in-formational and in-formed subsystem that is contemporary medicine and pharmacology is fascinating. That this subsystem would be closely connected and coherent with the global in-formation paradigm is extremely convincing. It is perfectly in line with the discoveries and the development of the fundamental sciences since the last century, even if mainstream medicine seems not to be aware of it yet. Now the time has come to update the official position of the medical and pharmacological systems in accordance with the advance of the major fields of science, especially physics. It is absurd that the interpretation of mainstream medicine should still be anchored in the state of knowledge of a century ago. Could this puzzling delay be connected with the strong conditioning of the academic world with the interests of Big Pharma? We do not know. For certain, Laszlo's and Biava's interpretation of the health/disease subsystem is perfectly in line with the vision of informational medical disciplines such as homeopathy, acupuncture, and bioresonance. These disciplines are not easily accepted by mainstream medicine and the Western academic environment. This is not the case in countries such as India and China, where homeopathy and acupuncture are highly valued and supported both by governments and universities.

Biava's research offers incontrovertible confirmation regarding the role of information in medicine. He discovered that the organogenesis phase in the genesis of the embryo is free of the danger of malignant tumors. Is this strange? Not so, really. The rationality of phylogenesis tells us that every new life must be protected so as to reach at least a basic level of development. Thus it makes sense that in the process of embryogenesis cancer cells should be ineffective. Biava's genius is to understand this process and to use the "tumor free" cells of the embryo to "remind" the cells of the living organism of their ontogenetic function. The clinical in vitro and in vivo studies reported in this book demonstrate that the information code in embryogenesis can in many cases eliminate cancer cells and rebalance the organism so as to prevent their replication and spread. It is astonishing to note that the cancer-preventing cells are those of the tiny Zebrafish embryo. This confirms the basic tenet of this book: that everything in the world is connected, and all healthy things are integrated.

A further demonstration that everything in the world is coherently connected is the fact that two great scientists have written an extraordinary work in perfect symbiosis. I trust that the evidence they produced will induce a positive shift in the thinking of everyone who reads this extraordinary treatise.

References

1. Mohan, V. *Liver cancer* (Hepatocellular carcinoma). https://Medicinenet .com.
2. *World Cancer Report 2014*. World Health Organization. 2014: Chapters 5.6 and 1.1.
3. *World Cancer Report 2014*. World Health Organization. 2014: Chapter 1.1. ISBN 9283204298. ISBN 9283204298.
4. GDB Collaborators. Global, regional, and national life expectancy, all-cause mortality, and cause-specific mortality for 249 causes of death, 1980–2015: a systematic analysis for the Global Burden of Disease Study. 2015. *Lancet*. 388 (10053): 1459–1544. DOI: http://dx.doi.org/10.1016 /S0140-6736(16)31012–1.

5. *World Cancer Report 2014*. World Health Organization. 2014: Chapter 5.6.

6. National Cancer Institute. Cancer Stat Facts: Liver and Intrahepatic Bile Duct Cancer. Seer.cancer.gov.

7. Richard Feynman. Quoted in: Simon Singh. How a big idea is born. *New Scientist*. 4 December 2004; 184(2476): 23.

8. Merchant C. The violence of impediments. *Isis*. 2008; 99:731–760. Available at: Nature.Berkeley.edu.

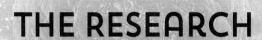

PART TWO

◎

THE RESEARCH

The Scientific Papers of Biava, et al.

INTRODUCTION

In part one we described the fundamental concept that underlies the promise of a new era in the history of healing and medicine and presented the discovery that is both a confirmation of the validity of this concept and a practical and beneficial breakthrough in its application. Now part two offers a pragmatic follow-up to these considerations. It is intended primarily for medical researchers and practitioners, but it is not without direct interest also to lay persons.

The same as part one, the purpose of the material presented in part two is twofold. On the one hand, it is to disclose the biophysical and biological specifics of the medical breakthrough, enabling practicing physicians to apply it in full knowledge of its scientific basis. On the other, the information communicated here is propaedeutic to opening the full potentials of the breakthrough, so as to usher in a new and beneficial era in the history of medicine and the art of healing. This is much needed, because the challenge to healing and medicine remains critical: despite great advances in the biochemical applications of contemporary medicine, tumoral and other chronic degenerative diseases remain rampant. However, the potentials of the new discovery are enormous. Creative researchers could find new applications of the discovery and find further areas and research domains to which the discovery could be extended.

Practical application and creative development are twin aspects of the challenge of information medicine to medical research and practice. They are priority domains both of contemporary medical science, and of therapeutic practice.

We hope that the scientific papers assembled in this part will prove to be of value to researchers and to practitioners in responding to the challenge and will help to usher in a much needed bright era in the maintenance of health and the healing of disease.

EDITORIALS

The two editorials included in this section offer overviews of new treatment possibilities, following close on the heels of rapid advances at the cutting edge of biochemical research into cell proliferation and differentiation. The new and ever-growing insight into the workings of stem cells led to a greater understanding of the behavior of tumor cells that exhibit similar characteristics and led to the discovery of practical ways of healing, or at least slowing, invasive cancerous growths. These are promising results for the treatment of a variety of other chronic diseases.

Complex Therapeutical Approaches to Complex Diseases

From *Current Pharmaceutical Biotechnology,* 2015, Volume 16, Number 9

Guest Editor: Pier Mario Biava

This article represents the editorial of a special issue of the journal Current Pharmaceutical Biotechnology, *whose title and subject were chosen by Biava as Guest Editor. This special issue consists of various articles, some of which are written by Biava and his collaborators, and other papers by various researchers in different parts of the world. The editorial illustrates the content of this special issue that describes the change of scientific paradigm needed to treat complex diseases such as cancer, chronic inflammatory, and degenerative diseases. The reductionist approach in addressing these complex pathologies reveals all its limitations, as shown by the poor clinical results obtained using this approach. Hence the need to tackle these diseases by adopting a complex and holistic approach.*

In the last decades the enormous advances in genetics and biology have made clear that cancer is a very complex disease sustained by many genetic and epigenetic alterations. They activate a great deal of pathological molecular pathways governing relevant physiological processes. In 2000 Hanahan and Weinberg identified six hallmarks of cancer diseases: 1) self-sufficiency in growth signals, 2) insensitivity to antigrowth signals, 3) limitless replicative potential, 4) ability to evade apoptosis, 5) support to angiogenesis, 6) invasion of tissue and ability to give metastasis. In addition, the lost differentiation of cancer cells was proposed recently by Biava P. M. (*Current Medicinal Chemistry* 2014) to the hallmarks of Hanahan and Weinberg.

Moreover, it was demonstrated that for normal cells to become cancerous, transformation also depends on a complex network of surrounding micro-environmental signals from cell-to-cell "cross-talking" or from soluble extracellular factors. For example, it has been demonstrated that inflammatory cells can sustain, instead of fighting tumor growth. Thus, the whole context is decisive in determining cell fate in line with a complex view of cell biology.

The current special issue describes why chronic diseases, including not only cancer, but also the metabolic syndrome, chronic inflammation, chronic degenerative diseases, etc. make diagnosis, prevention, and targeted therapeutic treatment particularly difficult. Recognition that chronic inflammation may induce genetic, neuro-endocrine, immune, and metabolic changes in a series of diseases is useful for designing new ways for prevention and treatment. A new approach may include reprogramming suppressive immune cells and pro-inflammatory mediators factors, restoring in this way the balance of neuro-endocrine-immune and metabolic network systems disrupted by chronic inflammation.

Differentiation factors, reprogramming therapies and immunotherapy are innovative biological means with more systemic approaches to cancer and chronic degenerative diseases treatment. In particular this special issue records some articles that highlight how growth and differentiation factors taken from a Zebrafish embryo could address the fate of normal and pathological (stem) cells. In fact, these factors taken during the early developmental stage of a Zebrafish embryo may represent a useful tool to enhance stem cell expression of multipotency and activate both telomerase-dependent and telomerase-independent antagonists of cell senescence. On the contrary, these factors taken during the late developmental stages decrease cell viability and direct cells toward senescence. This strategy did not require cumbersome gene manipulation through viral vector mediated gene transfer, or expensive synthetic chemistry. This data shows for the first time that it is possible to direct human mesenchymal stem cells toward different and opposite directions, tuning in specific, physiological ways the regulation of different genes. This is possible only when the specific networks of factors are sufficiently complex because single substances are not able to obtain any significant results.

These data lead us to consider a major shift in scientific paradigm (from reductionism to complexity) for preparing new treatments for chronic degenerative diseases. In fact, these diseases entail unexpected degrees of complexity and disregulation, making the single-molecule-to-specific-target paradigm totally obsolete and inadequate. Rather, only a systemic approach can be envisioned as a successful strategy to deal with such complexity. It is believed that time is ready for a "trans-disciplinary approach" in the treatment of degenerative diseases so that a new culture of collaboration can promote many important innovations and new therapeutic approaches.

Reprogramming of Normal and Cancer Stem Cells

From *Current Pharmaceutical Biotechnology*, 2011, Volume 12, Number 5

Guest Editor: Pier Mario Biava

This paper represents the editorial of a special issue of the journal Current Pharmaceutical Biotechnology, *whose title and subject were chosen by Biava as Guest Editor. This issue consists of fifteen articles, some of which were written by Biava and collaborators, and others by researchers of various scientific institutions. The editorial illustrates the content of this special issue.*

Over the last decade there has been an exponential rise in our understanding of the biochemical mechanisms controlling cell proliferation and differentiation. While the four transcription factors Oct4, Sox2, Klf4, and cMyc have shown to be sufficient to induce pluripotency in fibroblasts, there has in addition been much research into the mechanisms and pathways of cell differentiation and the specific properties of stem cells, namely their plasticity and capacity for trans-differentiation. These studies have allowed progress at a very fundamental level, with the prospect of further progress—until recent years quite unimaginable—in the field of reparative, regenerative, and transplant medicine. In fact, from the present time, the genetic engineering production of regulatory factors identified through such research, has allowed the production of new tissues and a new category of cell therapy products, in which the main biological action is carried out by cells or tissues, albeit in the presence of organic or inorganic matrices or coatings. Examples of this type of product are anti-tumor vaccines, in vitro cultivated skin, products made of structural and cellular elements for the reconstruction of bones, cartilages, teeth, etc.

From the best, most analytical and detailed characterization of stem cells, then, it has become clear that some tumor cell behaviors—that have a crucial role in determining their malignity—can be attributed to the presence of cells with characteristics similar to those of stem cells. The field of cancer research is consequently also witnessing a surge in studies designed to identify the metabolic pathways common to tumor and stem cells. This will in turn cast light on which micro-environment factors can direct these pathways toward differentiation and induce cancerous cells to behave less aggressively. From this point of view, over recent years there has been a lively return to studies that were very significant in the 70s and 80s, on the role of the embryonic micro-environment in conditioning tumor cell behavior toward normal phenotypes. This research is now underway, and will in all probability lead to important results over the next few years. Against this background, this special issue on "Reprogramming of Normal and Cancer Stem Cells" focuses on research in terms of conditioning the fate of normal and tumor stem cells with a view to new prospects for the therapies. The issue therefore begins with articles covering the possibility of reprogramming normal stem cells, including through use of biomaterials, and goes on to consider what characteristics of tumor stem cells can allow them to be identified and studied. This is followed by a series of further articles illustrating the role of the micro-environment in conditioning the fate of a tumor cell. A number of metabolic pathways characterizing and common to both stem and tumor cells are examined, in order to gain a better understanding of the possibilities of conditioning the fate of both cell types; in addition, the role played by infectious and inflammatory diseases in the genesis of tumor diseases is also considered.

Today, in fact, we know that inflammatory processes can support rather than hinder tumor growth, and also that pro-inflammatory cytokines can promote tumor proliferation, inhibiting the cell pathways that are able to block the neoplastic growth. The special issue goes on with a series of articles taking a close look at the specific role played by the micro-environment in conditioning the destiny of the tumor stem cells present in some tumors, for example breast and retinoblastoma tumor, and the role played by the use of normal stem cells in treating disorders such as hematological diseases. One article also considers the risks run by some reprogramming techniques: for example, creating embryo cells via parthenogenesis can give rise to tumors. The issue continues with various articles illustrating in close detail the role of the embryonic micro-environment in conditioning the destiny of tumor cells. In this context, one review takes a look at general aspects, while others consider aspects that can help clarify the mechanisms underlying the capacity of factors of this type of micro-environment to reprogram a tumor cell. One mathematical model sets out from a description of the state of cell differentiation, making use of existing data from studies of tumor growth slowing, linked to the use of such factors, with the goal of shedding light on aspects such as fitness, dosage, and administration time for the differentiation factors on improvement in tumor inhibitory response.

Other articles illustrate a number of clinical cases of full regression of hepatocellular carcinomas in intermediate-advanced stages observed following administration of stem cell differentiation factors, and describe the molecular mechanisms that might explain these inhibitory responses on the tumor growth. It should be noted that the randomized and controlled clinical studies launched to date using stem cell differentiation factors are limited to patients with intermediate-advanced stage of hepatocellular carcinomas where other therapies were no longer possible. These factors are at present used only for hepatocellular carcinomas, since it has been demonstrated that substances capable of slowing one tumor's growth may be inefficacious for another type. Finally, it is important to note that research into the possibility of reprogramming normal and tumor stem cells requires a complex approach to the issue. In fact, the problem requires the study of networks of substances and genes involved in the reprogramming phase, demanding skills in a variety of different areas of research, not simply of medical/biological, but also mathematical/computational and modeling, in view of the complexity and non-linearity of the processes being studied.

A paradigm shift is underway, and the future will witness our engagement in increasing numbers of scientific studies requiring cross-disciplinary skills. The new paradigm and the new ideas were well understood many years ago by Professor John Klavins, who has been a long-time President of the International Academy of Tumor Marker Oncology. Professor Klavins has always sustained my studies on reprogramming cancer cells, though the possibility of controlling tumor growth by using reprogramming factors was not considered realistic at the time I began studying it. I wish to dedicate the following reports to my friend John Klavins.

THE PRINCIPAL REPORTS

Cancer and Cell-Differentiation: A Model to Explain Malignancy

Journal of Tumor Marker Oncology, Fall 2002, Volume 17, Number 3

Pier Mario Biava, Daniele Bonsignorio

The article below is one of several articles in a special issue of the Journal of Tumor Marker Oncology, *the scientific official journal of the International Academy of Tumor Marker Oncology. This special issue contains scientific articles written by Biava et al., and the article below is the first article in the issue. It describes a model of cancer, the result of previous research carried out by Biava et al. in the laboratory. In this model tumor cells are described as cancer stem-like cells, which can be reprogrammed using the factors isolated from the embryo micro-environment.*

Introduction

The evidence obtained from studying the interactions between tumor cells and embryonic tissues suggests that tumor development in an embryo is reduced or suppressed when the processes of differentiation are in progress.[1,2]

In fact, the administration of known carcinogens in the course of cell differentiation in an embryo causes malformations in offspring, but not tumor induction. Once organogenesis is complete, the frequency of tumor induction rises with a concomitant decrease in the rate of malformations.[3,4,5]

These findings could indicate that cancer can be viewed as a developmental deviation susceptible to being controlled by regulators of cells differentiation.

On the basis of this background some experiments on animals were made. These previous experiments have demonstrated that factors present during cell differentiation are able to stop or delay tumor growth in animals. These factors are present in the pregnant uterus of mammals[6] and in the embryos of ovipari.[7] More recent experiments in vitro showed that pregnant pig and mouse uterus extracts slow down the proliferation rate of several established human tumor cell lines.[8] It was clarified that the abnormal growth of cell clones during embryo organogenesis in mammals is prevented by low-molecular weight substances present in pregnant uterus microenvironment. In fact a 5kDa fraction isolated in our laboratory from the pregnant uterus of mammals, named "Life-Protecting Factor," inhibited the cell proliferation curves of all treated human tumor cell lines as well as the crude pregnant uterus extracts. Therefore, the interactions between mother and embryo seem to be important for the normal development of the embryo and for preventing a pathological cell growth. The embryo itself seems to prevent the abnormal multiplication of tumor cells. In fact it was demonstrated that different tumor cell lines responded with a significant slowing of the proliferation when treated with extracts taken during the stages of cell differentiation, while no slowing effect was observed when they were treated with the extracts taken from a merely multiplicative stage.[9]

Thus, cell differentiation is a key process in understanding the behavior of both normal and tumor cells. The fact that embryonic development and tumorigenesis are closely correlated is now accepted: they both share several pathways and molecules, which are able to regulate some important genes of the cell cycle. In fact, the main effect of the in vitro treatment of tumor cell lines with the extracts of the oviparous embryos is the activation of p53 expression, as observed by immuno-histochemical and flow cytometry techniques after the treatment of different tumor cell lines with the extracts of fish embryos.[7] In addition we record in another article of this issue of the journal the induction of a post-translational regulation of pRb by the Zebrafish embryonic extracts, which is probably responsible for the observed slowing down of the kidney adenocarcinoma proliferation curves in vitro. Embryonic differentiation and tumorigenesis, although they share several metabolic pathways, seem to be opposite processes: the same molecules, which cause cell differentiation in the embryo, seem to be able to oppose the cancer growth. In order to elucidate the mechanisms involved in these two different processes, it is necessary to illustrate an outline and a model of embryonic differentiation and cancerogenesis.

An Outline and a Model of Embryonic Differentiation

Shortly after fertilization, generally in the middle-blastula-gastrula period, the processes of differentiation begin. There are three postulates of cell differentiation:

- Every cell nucleus contains the complete genome established in the fertilized egg. In molecular terms the DNAs of all differentiated cells are identical.
- The unused genes in the differentiated cells are not destroyed or mutated, and they retain the potential for being expressed.
- Only a small percentage of genome is expressed in each differentiated cell and a portion of the RNA synthesized is specific for that cell type.

Briefly, the differentiation, which leads pluripotent embryonic stem cells to specialization, consists in a differential regulation of genes that restricts the expressed genome. The gene configurations of the cells, which rise after each stage of differentiation, differ from the progenitors for some thousands of expressed genes.

Regulators are generally factors that cooperate in a network, and this network promotes and controls the differentiation of each cell type. All cells communicate with each other through this network.

Cell differentiation is a very complex process that takes place at different levels:

A) a differential gene transcription that regulates how the nuclear genes are transcripted into RNA

B) a selective nuclear RNA processing that regulates how the transcript RNAs get into cytoplasm to become messenger RNAs

C) a selective messenger RNA translation that regulates how messenger RNAs in cytoplasm get translated into proteins

D) a differential modification of proteins that regulates how proteins are allowed to function in the cells

Transcription factors are very important in controlling the differential expression of genes, but in eukariotes selective nuclear RNAs' processes are more important. These selective processes clarify how the same gene can produce two different proteins in different cells or in the same cell at different times. Besides selective degradation, otherwise selective stabilization of messenger RNA is responsible for further specifications of proteins.

Today we have a dynamic vision of the regulation of gene expression. We think that a gene is not an independent and autonomous center of control of the synthesis of proteins; a gene is also controlled directly or indirectly by synthesized proteins.

Certainly, the interactions between nucleus and cytoplasm and between cytoplasm and microenvironment are so wide that they constitute a marvelous example of complexity. Developing embryo is an excellent example of what is called "complex adaptive systems." In fact an embryo: 1) is a network of many cells acting in parallel, 2) has many levels of organization that are constantly revising and rearranging, 3) has an implicit prediction encoded in its genes and

4) is always in transition and is characterized by perpetual novelty.

Cell differentiation can be better understood by a model described here, which is consistent with the real situation. In this model the number of final gene configurations of cells in the human body (number of types of completely differentiated cells) can be predicted, if we retain that each kind of progenitor cells produces three different daughter cells (different gene configurations) and that there are five stages of differentiation. This corresponds to the real situation: in fact the embryo, after segmentation (morula), differentiates in three layers: ectoderm, endoderm, and mesoderm. Gametes differentiate in a different pathway than somatic cells. After gastrulation, there are four more stages of cell differentiation. For example, on the basis of precise data about some cell lines, like hematopoietic cells, the stages of differentiation are: a) stem cell stage, b) committed stem cell stage, c) differentiating cell stage, d) differentiated cell stage. If we include the ectodermal, endodermal, and mesodermal cell lines, the stages of differentiation are five. Therefore, the mathematical formula to calculate the number of differentiated cells is:

$$N = 3^5$$

The result is 243, which is the number of the various somatic differentiated cells. To calculate the final number of the differentiated cells we have to add the number of gametes. The sexual cells are 5 in men (spermatogonium, spermatocyte of the first order, spermatocyte of the second order, spermatid, spermatozoon) and 4 in women (ovogonium, ovocyte of the first order, ovocyte of the second order, egg cell). The final result is 252, which is the number of the different kinds of cells in humans.

Cancer as Undifferentiated Mutated Cells:
A Model to Explain Malignancy

Tumoral transformation of normal cells is a process relying on a minimal number of stochastic mutational events, comprised between 4 and 7.[10] If mutations are introduced into normal cells in a non-stochastic manner, i.e., triggering at precise genes, that number is even reduced.[11] Preferential targets of these mutations are genes encoding for key-role effectors of cell cycle regulation and cell signaling, and for growth factors and their receptors; mutations are either gain-of-function, in case of proto-oncogenes, or loss-of-function, in case of tumor suppressor genes.

Anyway, defining the tumoral transformation of a cell simply as an outcome of a sum of gene mutations may be reductive. For normal cells to turn to cancerous, transformation depends also on a complex network of surrounding microenvironmental signals, coming from cell-to-cell "cross-talking" or from soluble extracellular factors. For example, it has been demonstrated that fibroblasts adjacent to prostate epithelium carcinoma cells are able to direct tumor progression,[12] that stromal neighbor cells are able to promote malignant transformation of immortalized keratinocytes by releasing proliferative stimuli,[13] and that inflammatory cells can sustain instead of fight tumor growth.[14] Even pro-inflammatory cytokines were shown to promote cancer cell proliferation by inhibiting tumor suppression pathways.[15] Thus, the whole context is decisive in determining cell fate according to a "heterotypic" view of cell biology, as it was called in a recent review.[16]

According to this view, defining tumorigenesis as a microevolutive process is no more a hazard. A cancer cell acquires, as consequence of this process, some capabilities: 1) self-sufficiency in growth signals, 2) insensitivity to antigrowth signals, 3) capability in evading apoptosis, 4) limitless replicative potential, 5) capability in sustaining angiogenesis, 6) capability in invading tissues and in metastasizing. The acquisition of the enumerated capabilities during the course of tumor progression is usually the consequence of a great variability on the way that cells take to becoming malignant. Nonetheless the hypothesis advanced here is that independent of how the steps in these genetic pathways are arranged, the development of all types of human tumor cells is governed by a final common process. Some authors define "early crisis" and "genetic catastrophe" of a cell as steps that enable an evolving population of premalignant cells to reach malignancy.[17] These crises, during which a telomere dysfunction and a DNA damage take place, give rise to different possibilities: 1) cells die, or 2) cells survive after each crisis. The final results are adaptive responses and telomere maintenance in the case of cells survival. Those surviving malignant cells have a) not only increased the level of telomerase, but b) have also activated proto-oncogenes or oncogenes, c) produce growth factors, d) are insensitive to anti-growth signals, e) have several surface antigens, also known as oncofetal antigens, maintained during philogeny, most of which have been identified in the last 30 years.[18-27] In other terms the cells that survive a genetic instability period become malignant through the achievement of a new stable genes configuration very similar to those present in an embryo during the periods of multiplication.

In fact, cancer cells and embryonic cells share some molecular pathways and their key-role effectors: for example, the APC/b catenin/TCF/Wnt pathway[28,29] and the Hedgehog/Smoothened/Patched pathway.[30] Whereas in the embryonic development these pathways lead cells to successful differentiation, in tumorigenesis their mutated counterparts lead cells to a constant multiplication. This happens because a cancer cell is an undifferentiated cell, in which the mutations present in its genome prevent the cell from completing the whole program of differentiation and development. It is stopped in a step of multiplication, comprised between two stages of differentiation. A cancer cell can be defined as an "undifferentiated mutated cell," in which the program of differentiation and multiplication are uncoupled. It is like a computer in loop, repeating always the same instructions. Cancer is an example of deterministic chaos. It is a branching process, that conduces a cell, since it does not die, to a rampant genetic instability: the final attractor is a new stable "gene configuration" similar to that present in an embryo during the steps of multiplication, comprised between two stages of differentiation. In this hypothesis, considering the model of cell differentiation previously mentioned, the number of different types of cancer derived from somatic cells can be predicted by the formula:

$$N = 3 + 3^2 + 3^3 + 3^4 = 120$$

In order to calculate the final number of different kinds of tumors, it is necessary to add the number of tumors coming from sexual cells and from different embryonic tissues (teratocarcinoma, embryonic carcinoma, corioncarcinoma). Therefore the final amount of all different kinds of tumor is about 130. With regard to malignancy it has to be considered that the most aggressive tumors are represented by cells with "gene configurations" present at early stages of differentiation that carry out the program of multiplication with impressive speed. Besides, it has to be remembered that the current classification of tumors is redundant, because it does not consider that the most malignant types of tumors are constituted by kinds of cells, which have the same "gene configurations." Finally it has to be remembered that some types of tumors are constituted by different cell clones with "gene configurations" coming from different stages of differentiation.

The Regulation of Cancer Growth:
A Model of Complexity

The model of cancer as proposed above is not merely theoretical, but relies on the results of the experiments performed in our lab. Those experiments have shown that molecular factors present during precise stages of cell differentiation are able to inhibit tumor growth. This was demonstrated both *in vivo* on Lewis cancer and *in vitro* on several human tumor cell lines. On the contrary, substances present during merely proliferative stages are not effective in delaying the growth curves of several types of tumors. Thus, cell differentiation is a key process for elucidating the behavior of both undifferentiated normal and tumor cells. The mechanisms by which the events of cell differentiation take place rely on a multigenic regulation, so that a more differentiated cell differs from a less differentiated one for the expression of a great number of genes. Furthermore, it has to be marked that, according to the above model, tumor cells have lost an important portion of the program of cell differentiation in a progressive manner.

So said, if ultimately the aim is not the destruction of the tumor cell, but its regulation, it is clear that the goal can be achieved only by providing the cell with all the factors that are able to bring it to differentiation. These factors can be found, but only when life is forming. In fact, during organogenesis the whole repertoire of regulatory molecules is present, which includes 1) DNA transcriptional factors; 2) nuclear RNA selection factors; 3) mRNA translational factors; 4) post-translational protein regulatory factors. As shown, it is possible to use these factors for the genic regulation of tumor cells. A p53-mediated transcriptional regulation and a pRb post-translational regulation were demonstrated, depending on the type of tumor. Thus, it was demonstrated that it is possible to regulate tumor cells, by-passing mutations that give rise to malignancy. This happens only when the network of differentiation is complete enough.

From this point of view it is necessary to focus on the microenvironments and the networks that constitute the biological structures, rather than the single subjects of punctual mechanisms. This does not mean that the research of molecular mechanisms should be left behind, only that there is a need to bring the single partial mechanisms to a synthesis. Indeed, the difficulty of bridging the gap to a new scientific paradigm, that is, shifting our views from reductionism to complexity, has been the main hindrance to a deeper and more complete knowledge of cancer. While studies and researches on stem cells differentiation are proceeding worldwide, the scientific community is ready to accept a change of paradigm. In fact, those studies will be able to show that the mechanisms of differentiation depend on specific differentiating networks. The embryonic microenvironment during precise stages of development is fundamental not only for the differentiation of the normal stem cells but also for the differentiation of tumor cells. The embryo, during organogenesis, is never affected by carcinogenetic processes because, while the life program is under transcription, systems of correction in case of mutations are also active. In fact, it was demonstrated that during cell differentiation the administration of known carcinogens fails to induce the growth of tumors, perhaps because the genome control system is always working.

Recent studies claim that p53 function in the embryo is to prevent malformations, so that some authors have called p53 "guardian of the babies," as a gene that suppresses the onset of malformations. Anyway, when the stress is too severe and the mutations are too numerous, p53 is no longer able to repair DNA and provokes apoptosis in all cells. These processes also occur in tumor cells when p53 is active. In these regards, tumor cells are similar to mutated embryonic cells.

References

1. Einhorn L. *Oncodev Biol Med* (1982), 4:219–229.
2. Lakshmi MS & Sherbert GV. Embryonic and Tumor Cells Interactions. Karger. Basel 1974: 380–399.
3. Brent RL. *Teratology* (1980), 21:281–298.
4. Rice JM. *Teratology* (1973), 8:113–125.
5. Tomatis L, Mohr V. Transplacental Carcinogenesis. *IARC Sci. Publ. no.4 Lyon* 1973.
6. PM Biava, A Fiorito, C Negro & M Mariani. *Cancer Lett* (1988), 41:265–270.
7. PM Biava & A Carluccio. *J Tumor Marker Oncol* (1997), 4:9–15.
8. PM Biava, D Bonsignorio & M Hoxha. *J Tumor Marker Oncol* (2000), 15:223–233.
9. PM Biava, D Bonsignorio & M Hoxha. *J Tumor Marker Oncol* (2001), 16:195–201.
10. Renan MJ. *Mol Carcinogenesis* (1993), 7:139–146.
11. Hahn WC, Counter CM, Lundberg AS, Beijersbergen RL, Brooks MW & Weinberg RA. *Nature* (1999), 400:464–468.
12. Olumi AF, Grossfeld GD, Hayward SW, Carroll, PR, Tlsty TD & Cunha GR. *Cancer Res* (1999), 59:5002–5011.
13. Skobe M & Fusenig NE. *Proc Natl Acad Sci USA* (1998), 95:1050–1055.
14. Coussens LM, Raymond WW, Bergers G, Laig-Webster M, Behrendtsen O, Werb Z, Cughey GH & Hanahan D. *Genes Dev* (1998), 13:1382–1397.

15. Hudson JD, Shoaibi MA, Maestro R, Carnero A, Hannon GJ & Beach DH. *J Exp Med* (1999), 190:1375–1382.
16. Hanahan D & Weinberg RA. *Cell* (2000), 100:57–70.
17. Chin L, Artandi SE, Shen Q, Tam A, Lee S-L, Gottlieb GJ, Greider CW & DePinho RA. *Cell* (1999), 97:527–538.
18. LeMevel BP & Wells SA Jr. *Nature (New Biol)*, 244 (136): 183–4 (1973).
19. Shah LP, Rees RC & Baldwin RW. *Br J Cancer*, 33 (6): 577–83 (1976).
20. Steele G Jr & Sjogren HO. *Int J Cancer*, 14 (4): 435–444 (1974).
21. Ting C-C & Grant JP. *J Natl Cancer Inst*, 56 (2): 401–4 (1976).
22. Ting C-C, Sanford KK & Price FM. *In Vitro*, 14 (2): 207–11 (1978).
23. Menard S, Colnaghi MI & Della Porta G. *Tumori*, 63 (4): 359–66 (1977).
24. Woo J & Cater DB. *Biochem J*, 128 (5): 1273–84 (1972).
25. Wahlström T, Linder W & Saksela E. *Acta Pathol Microbiol Scand*, 81 (6): 768–774 (1973).
26. Medawar P & Hunt R. *Cancer Res*, 36 (9): 3453–4 (1976).
27. Zhang S, Sell S, Livingston PO, Klavins JV. *J Tumor Marker Oncol*, 12:52 (1997).
28. M Peifer & P Polakis. *Science* (2000), 287:1606–1609.
29. P Polakis. *Genes Dev* (2000), 14:1837–1851.
30. PW Ingham. *Curr Opin Gen Dev* (1998), 8:88–94.

Stem Cell Differentiation Stage Factors from Zebrafish Embryo: A Novel Strategy to Modulate the Fate of Normal and Pathological Human (Stem) Cells

Current Pharmaceutical Biotechnology, 2015, Volume 16, Number 9: 782–92.

Pier Mario Biava, Silvia Canaider, Federica Facchin, Eva Bianconi, Liza Ljungberg, Domenico Rotilio, Fabio Burigana, and Carlo Ventura

This article is important because it describes the different functions of the epigenetic code that have been studied and analyzed in a long research process. In addition to the way in which the cancer cells can be reprogrammed, it also illustrates how it is possible to prevent aging and neurodegeneration and to ameliorate the clinical results in psoriasis patients. The article shows how the current scientific paradigm, based on reductionism, needs to be changed in depth, as it highlights how the results obtained in the prevention of complex pathologies, as these described in the article, are only possible when the information transferred to DNA from the epigenetic code is complete and redundant.

Introduction

Current medical literature acknowledges that embryonic microenvironment is able to suppress tumor development during cell differentiating processes.[1,2] Administration of carcinogenic substances during organogenesis leads in fact to embryonic malformations, but not to offspring tumor growth. However, administration of carcinogenic substances after complete organogenesis causes a rise in offspring tumor development.[3,4,5] This data indicates that cancer can be considered as a deviation in normal development that can be controlled by factors in embryonic microenvironment during the differentiating stages. Furthermore, it has been demonstrated that teratoma differentiates into normal tissues once implanted in the embryo.[6]

Recently, it has been shown that implantation of melanoma cells into Zebrafish embryos does not result in tumor development, while in the adult animal, a tumor is formed.[7] Moreover, injection of melanoma cells in Zebrafish extra-embryonic membranes originated Zebrafish neuronal cells. This demonstrates that cancer cells can differentiate in normal tissues when implanted in embryos.[8] In addition, it was demonstrated that other tumors, including leukemia, liver, and breast tumor cells, can revert into a normal phenotype and/or differentiate into normal tissue when implanted in the embryo.[9,10,11,12]

The term "reprogramming" was initially introduced to identify the transformation of a normal adult somatic cell into an embryonic-like stem cell, into so-called induced pluripotent stem cells (iPS). The issue of cell reprogramming has now been extended to cancer (stem) cells to define any genetic or epigenetic intervention aimed at inducing differentiation of these cells into a normal phenotype and/

or forcing them to become terminally differentiating cells. These interventions focus on the role of the embryonic microenvironment in tumor reprogramming. Intriguingly, it is now evident that the molecular mechanisms underlying normal stem cell differentiation and embryonic development do not stop after birth but are still in part operating and remodeled throughout the adult life to maintain the self-identity and the interplay between tissues and organs. To this end, it has been shown that the transcription factor GATA4 is a critical regulator of both embryonic and postnatal heart development and morphogenic maintenance due to a fine tuning of its structural/regulatory domains.[13] Whereas the N-terminal domain of GATA4 is required for inducing cardiogenesis and for promoting postnatal cardiomyocyte survival, distinct residues and domains therein are necessary to mediate these effects.[13] Cardiogenic activity of GATA4 requires a 24-amino-acid (aa) region (aa 129 to 152) which is needed for transcriptional synergy and physical interaction with BAF60c. The same region is not essential for induction of endoderm or blood cell markers by GATA4, suggesting that it acts as a cell-type-specific transcriptional activation domain. On the other hand, a serine residue at position 105, which is a known target for mitogen-activated protein kinase (MAPK) phosphorylation, is necessary for GATA4-dependent cardiac myocyte survival and hypertrophy but is entirely dispensable for GATA4-induced cardiogenesis.[13]

A noteworthy example of morphogenetic flexibility is also provided by the existence of reverse pathways of transformation, from the postnatal stage back to an embryonic-like condition retaining the memory ability to re-differentiate backward to the same original phenotype. A vivid example of such flexibility is shown by the ability of post-natal cardiomyocytes to generate iPS cells with enhanced capacity toward cardiomyogenic re-differentiation.[14] Similarly, adult neurogenesis, a process of generating functional neurons from adult neural precursors, has been shown to occur throughout life in restricted brain regions in mammals, including the dentate gyrus of the hippocampus, the subventricular zone of the lateral ventricle, and the rostral migratory stream to the olfactory bulb.[15] This discovery is currently boosting emerging principles that have significant implications not only in stem cell biology, developmental neurobiology, and neural plasticity, but, remarkably, in disease mechanisms, including neurodegeneration.

Hence, a kind of memory/projection of the embryonic patterning may be conceived as a relevant background in tissue resident stem cells in the adulthood for the execution of self-healing and "learning" (acquirement of new knowledge) tasks. In this frame, degenerative diseases occurring in any organ (i.e., neurodegenerative diseases) may be viewed as a deviation from the normal potential of tissue resident stem cells to afford self-healing duties and the maintenance of tissue organ identity.

Akin to this perception, here we review several of our experimental findings over the past 20 years on the possibility to reprogram cancer cells *in vitro* as well as *in vivo*. In fact, we present results from controlled clinical studies on hepatocellular carcinoma at intermediate-advanced stage based on the treatment with Zebrafish stem cell differentiation stage factors (SCDSFs) taken during precise stages of stem cell differentiating processes.[16,17] We also report on our recent finding that the same SCDSFs obtained at early developmental stages acted as a major controller of stemness and senescence patterning in human adult adipose-derived stem cells.[18] Consistent with the concept of considering tissue degeneration a "flexible" deviation from a tissue identity program still entangled with embryogenetic memory, we show our recent findings on the ability of SCDSFs to prevent neurodegeneration in hippocampal cells of CA1 area in mice. Compounding the spectrum of exploitation of SCDSF potential for (stem) cell reprogramming, we recently succeeded in using Zebrafish embryo-extracts to reduce keratosis and ameliorate symptoms in patients affected by psoriasis,[19,20,21] a T-cell-dependent immune-mediated disease of the skin and joints. Such result is also rewarding due to (i) the recent detection of functional circadian clocks in most, if not all, skin cell types, (ii) the emergence of a close involvement of these circadian clocks in the control of

UVB-induced DNA damage and skin cancers, and (iii) the implication for the targeted modulation of stem-cell-mediated immunomodulatory action and control of aging processes.[22,23]

Role of SCDSFs in Cancer Cell Lines and in Mice Carcinoma Cells

In vitro effects of SCDSFs on different human tumor cell lines have been investigated in a number of studies.[24,25,26,27,28] Seven different human tumor cell lines (glioblastoma multiforme, melanoma, hepatocarcinoma, kidney adenocarcinoma, colon and breast adenocarcinoma, acute lymphoblastic and leukemia) were treated with factors taken from Zebrafish embryos at different developmental phases, specific of the beginning, intermediate and final embryonic differentiation stages. In general, a reduced growth rate was seen when tumor cells lines were treated with factors drawn during the different developmental stages, ranging from 73 percent reduction for the glioblastoma cells to 26 percent for the melanoma cells. No proliferative effects have been reported, except from a weak tumoral growth with factors extracted at a very early stage of embryonic development in which the differentiation processes did not begin, like morula stage. These data confirm the intuition that in the embryo, during the differentiating stages, there are networks of factors able to readdress tumoral cells toward a normal path. Those networks appear in the very first phases of the gastrulation, while they are absent in merely multiplicative stages.[24]

Several studies were carried out in order to unravel the molecular mechanisms involved in tumor growth inhibition mediated by Zebrafish embryonic extracts, showing that molecules that have a fundamental role in regulation of the cell cycle, such as p53 and retinoblastoma protein (pRb) were affected. More precisely, a p53 transcriptional regulation took place, highlighted by a considerable increase of the p53 protein expression in some of the tumor cell lines, such as the glioblastoma multiforme and the melanoma.[25] In other tumor cell lines, such as kidney adenocarcinoma, the growth reduction was due to changes in phosphorylation of pRb,[26] which is known to regulate transcription of E2F-1 and thereby control the cell cycle.

Moreover, apoptotic events as well as cell differentiation events were studied, in order to understand the consequences of cell cycle regulation in tumor cells induced by differentiation factors. The analysis was carried out on colon adenocarcinoma cells, showing activation of an apoptotic pathway dependent on p73, as well as an increase in the cell differentiation marker e-cadherin.[27]

Finally, in order to ascertain if SCDSFs could synergistically/ additively interact with 5-Fluorouracil (5-Fu), whole cell-count, flow-cytometry analysis and apoptotic parameters were recorded in human colon cancer cells (Caco-2) treated with SCDSFs 3 μg/ml in association or not with 5-Fu in the sub-pharmacological therapeutic range (0.01 mg/ml). Cell proliferation was significantly reduced by SCDSFs, meanwhile SCDSF+5-Fu leads to an almost complete growth-inhibition. SCDSFs produce a significant apoptotic effect, meanwhile the association with 5-Fu leads to an enhanced additive apoptotic rate at both 24 and 72 hours. SCDSFs alone and in association with 5-Fu trigger both the extrinsic and the intrinsic apoptotic pathways, activating caspase-8, -3 and -7. SCDSFs and 5-Fu alone exerted opposite effects on Bax and Bcl-xL proteins, meanwhile SCDSFs+5-Fu induced an almost complete suppression of Bcl-xL release and a dramatic increase in the Bax/Bcl-xL ratio. These data suggest that Zebrafish embryonic factors could improve chemotherapy efficacy by reducing anti-apoptotic proteins involved in drug-resistance processes.[28] Therefore, the molecular mechanisms underlying the tumor growth reduction seen after treatment with SCDSFs can be summarized as follows: the cell cycle stops in G1-S or G2-M phase, according to the tumor type, genetic damage repair and cell re-differentiation, or tumor cells apoptosis if reparation is not possible because of mutation gravity.

The effects of SCDSFs on tumor growth were also observed *in vivo* after subcutaneous injection of primary Lewis Lung Carcinoma cells into C57BL/6 female syngenic mice weighing 18–20 gr. A single cell suspension of tumor cells was prepared by mechanical dissociation of tumor mass: 50 μL of Dulbecco phosphate buffered saline (DPBS) containing 10^6 viable tumor cells were mixed with SCDSFs and used in the treated animals, while the control group received 50 mL of DPBS. The growth of the primary tumor was measured with calipers at different days after the injection, and the survival time was recorded. A highly significant difference was noted (p<0.001) between treated and control mice both in terms of primary tumor development and of the survival rate in favor of the treated mice.[29]

SCDSFs in Clinical Trials on
Intermediate-Advanced Hepatocellular Carcinoma (HCC)

From the 1st of January 2001 to the 31st of April 2004 a randomized controlled clinical trial was conducted on 179 patients affected by HCC in an intermediate-advanced stage. Since no further treatments were possible, a product fine-tuned on the basis of the above-mentioned studies was administered. The posology was 30 sublingual drops of the 50 percent epiboly Zebrafish embryo extract three times a day. The sublingual solution was chosen because the composition of the active fraction is composed of low molecular weight proteins (see the data about the protein analysis of SCDSFs on pages 109–111).

Objective tumor response, overall survival, and performance status have been evaluated. Results showed that 19.8 percent of the patients experienced a regression and 16 percent experienced a stabilization with an overall survival of more than 60 percent of the responsive patients after 40 months, compared to 10 percent of the non responsive patients.

A wide improvement of performance status has been registered in a great majority of patients (82.6 percent), also in those who experienced a progression of the disease.[16] A more recent study confirms the role of SCDSFs in determining complete response in primitive intermediate advanced liver cancer in 13.1 percent of patients.[17]

SCDSFs in Human Adipose-Derived Stem Cells (hASCs)

The possibility to address the fate of hASCs, isolated from a micro-fractured fat tissue obtained with a novel non-enzymatic method and device (Lipogems)[30], was explored by exposing them to SCDSFs.[18]

SCDSFs taken during the late developmental stages (20 somites and pharyngula stages) decreased cell viability and elicited caspase-3 mediated apoptosis. This effect did not involve *Bax* or *Bcl-2* transcription. This phenomenon has long been observed, as shown in the case of Bax-independent, caspase-3-related apoptosis induced by hepatocyte growth factor (HGF) in rat liver epithelial cells and recently confirmed in both malignant and normal cells.[31]

Unlike SCDSFs taken during the late developmental stages, SCDSFs taken during the early developmental stage (50 percent epiboly stage) did not induce hASC apoptosis, nor did it decrease cell viability. Indeed, SCDSFs of the early developmental stage were able to modulate the stem-cell expression of multipotency, enhancing the stemness genes *Oct-4, Sox-2,* and *c-Myc*. In addition to affecting stemness genes that maintain stem-cell identity,[32] SCDSFs also elicited transcriptional activation of two major mechanisms capable of counteracting stem-cell senescence, including the gene expression of TERT, the catalytic sub-unit of telomerase, and the gene transcription of *Bmi-1*. This is a member of the Polycomb and Trithorax families of repressors which acts as essential factors for self-renewal of adult stem cells, and as a key telomerase independent repressor of cell aging.[33]

Thus, this study showed that human stem cell exposure to SCDSFs taken during the early developmental stage of Zebrafish embryo may represent a useful tool to enhance stem-cell expression of multipotency and activate both telomerase-dependent and -independent antagonists of cell senescence. On the contrary SCDSFs taken during the late developmental stages decrease cell viability and induce cells toward senescence. This strategy did not require cumbersome gene manipulation through viral vector mediated gene transfer, or expensive synthetic chemistry. This data shows for the first time in the world that it is possible to induce human mesenchymal stem cells toward different and opposite directions, tuning in a specific, physiological way the regulation of different genes.

The Neuroprotective Role of SCDSFs

We present here, for the first time, some recent findings on the ability of SCDSFs to prevent neurodegeneration in hippocampal cells of CA1 area in mice.

In order to evaluate the neuroprotective effect of SCDSFs, murine hippocampal slices of the CA1 area were prepared and cultured as described by Gardoni et al.[34] and four Zebrafish embryo solutions were prepared as follows: A (50 percent epiboly plus tail bud stage extracts), B (5 somites stage), C (20 somites plus pharingula stage), and Mix ABC (a mixture of the three solutions A, B and C).[24]

Organotypic hippocampal slices were treated with N-Methyl-D-Aspartate (NMDA) 50 μM and 300 μM for 1 hour to induce mortality and a propidium iodide (PI) coloration was performed after 24 hours.[35] After fixing, the CA1 area was acquired and mortality was analyzed considering the average PI-fluorescence intensity, using as a term of comparison the maximum cell damage obtained by exposing the organotypic slices to NMDA. We first observed that treatment with NMDA 50 μM and 300 μM induced an increase of mortality of 47 percent and 139 percent respectively compared with the controls (p=0.002 and p=0.0002 respectively).

Then we evaluated the neuroprotective effect of SCDSFs after treatment with three toxic stimuli administered for 1 hour at the 14th day of culture: they were serum deprivation, NMDA 50 μM, and NMDA 300 μM. Analyses were performed 24 hours after treatments.

We noticed that treatment with the Mix ABC (dilution 1:100) subministrated together with each of the three toxic stimuli reduced in a significant manner the neuronal mortality caused by both serum deprivation and NMDA treatments. In fact SCDSFs significantly reduce the neuronal mortality caused by serum deprivation (-31.6 ± 6.2 percent, p=0.005) as shown in figure 1 (see page 106).

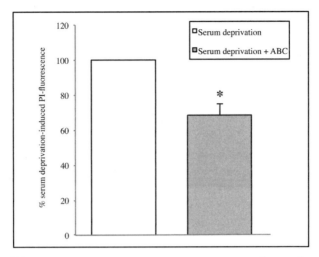

Figure 1. The effect of the Mix ABC on CA1 area cell mortality
after 1 hour of serum deprivation (*p=0.005)

Moreover, treatment with NMDA 50 μM significantly increases cell mortality compared with the controls (p=0.002), and SCDSFs significantly reduce the neuronal mortality caused by NMDA 50 μM treatment (p=0.01) as shown in figure 2.

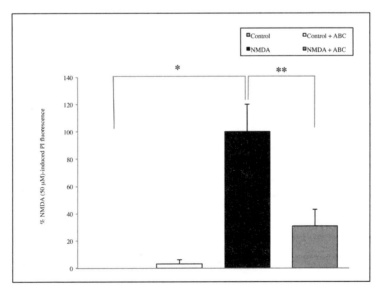

Figure 2. The effect of the Mix ABC on CA1 area cell mortality
after 1 hour NMDA 50 μM treatment (*p=0.002; **p=0.01)

Similarly, treatment with NMDA 300 μM significantly increases cell mortality compared with the controls (p=0.0002) and SCDSFs significantly reduce the neuronal mortality caused by NMDA 300 μM treatment (p=0.009) as shown in figure 3.

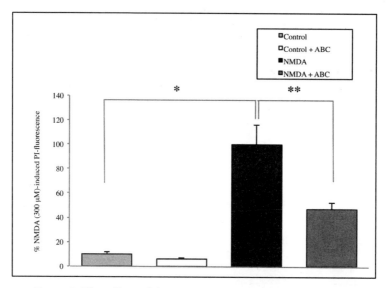

Figure 3. The effect of the Mix ABC on CA1 area cell mortality after 1 hour NMDA 300 μM treatment (*p=0.0002; **p=0.009)

Subsequently, the potential neuroprotective activities of A or B or C were investigated. Also in this case, the experiments showed a reduction in mortality overall for A extract, but results are not enough significant, neither in the serum deprivation group (figure 4) nor in the NMDA group (figure 5) (see page 108). Thus, the whole informational set with a redundance of differentiation stage factors is needed to produce an effective result.

Experimental Research and Clinical Studies on Psoriasis

We also investigated the anti-proliferative effects of SCDSFs by addressing the mitochondrial function (MTT assay) and cell nuclei distribution (Hoechst staining) in epidermal cell cultures stimulated with fetal calf serum (FCS) or epidermal growth factor (EGF). SCDSFs significantly

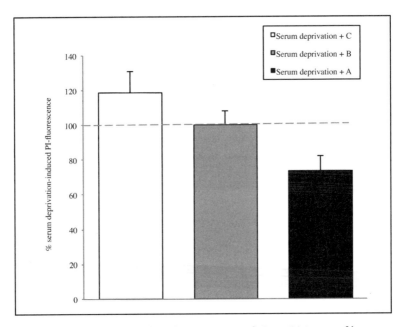

Figure 4. The effect of the single solutions A, B and C on CA1 area of hippocamp after 1 hour of serum deprivation. Values are expressed as percentage of samples treated with serum deprivation without SCDSFs.

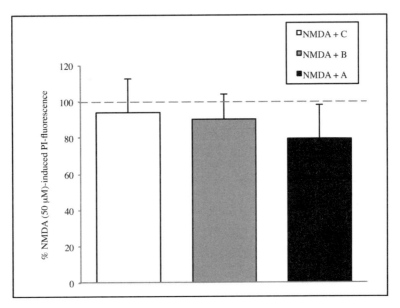

Figure 5. The effect of the single solutions A, B, and C on CA1 area of hippocamp after 1 hour of NMDA 50 μM treatment. Values are expressed as a percentage of samples treated with NMDA 50 μM without SCDSFs.

inhibited cell proliferation induced by either approach, although the effect was stronger in cells stimulated with FCS.[36] Three clinical trials were conducted to evaluate the efficacy in cases of psoriasis following the administration of a mix of all 5 Zebrafish embryo developmental stage extracts added with *Boswelia serrata*, 18-beta glycyrrhetic acid, *Zanthoxylum alatum*, 7-dehydro-cholesterol, and vitamin E. Results show 80 percent clinical objective improvements, with a reduction of keratosis and itch after 20–30 days from the beginning of the treatment.[19,20,21]

Protein Analysis of SCDSFs

To better know the content of the SCDSFs that we employed for our researches, we began to perform protein analysis of the extracts, and here we present our first results.

First, protein content of the five Zebrafish embryo extracts re-suspended in a glycero-alcoholic solution[18,24] was analyzed on a one-dimensional Sodium Dodecyl Sulphate-PolyAcrylamide Gel Electrophoresis (SDS-PAGE).[37] After Coomassie staining,[38] the protein amount was evaluated as pixel intensity, and relative abundances were expressed as a percentage of the total intensity. As shown in figure 6, in all five extracts, three main protein clusters are distinguishable according

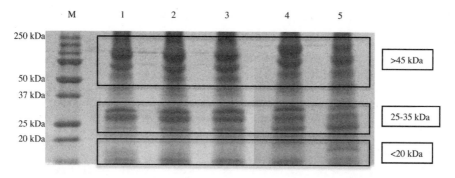

Figure 6. Representative 12 percent SDS-PAGE gel of Zebrafish embryo extracts resuspended in a glycero-alcoholic solution. Lanes: M) Broad-range protein molecular weight markers (in kDa); 1) 50 percent epiboly stage proteins; 2) tail bud stage proteins; 3) 5 somites stage proteins; 4) 20 somites stage proteins; 5) pharingula stage proteins.

to their molecular weight; i.e., over 45 kDa, around 25–35 kDa, and less than 20 kDa. In any case, the relative protein abundance is different among the five samples.

At the beginning of the gastrula period (50 percent epiboly stage, Lane 1), the higher molecular weight cluster (> 45 kDa) represents the 45.8 percent of the bands' intensity; this relative abundance is quite stable at the end of the gastrula period (tail bud stage, Lane 2) with a peak at the beginning of the segmentation, 46.1 percent (5 somites, Lane 3), while at the middle-late segmentation (20 somites, Lane 4 and pharyngula, Lane 5) this percentage composition decreases until the 43.9 percent.

The 25–35 kDa protein cluster abundance is quite stable in the gastrula period (Lanes 1 and 2), around 25.5 percent, while during the segmentation (Lanes 3, 4 and 5) it decreases until the 22.6 percent. At the beginning of the gastrula period (50 percent epiboly stage, Lane 1) the lowest molecular weight cluster (less then 20 kDa) represent the 28.5 percent; the cluster abundance is quite similar among the end gastrulation and early segmentation (Lanes 2 and 3) (29.4 percent) while at the end of the gastrulation stages (20 somites, Lane 4, and pharingula, Lane 5) the percentage increases until 33.5 percent.

Then, all the proteins extracted from the earliest Zebrafish developmental investigated stage (50 percent epiboly) were identified by using a liquid chromatography–mass spectrometry (LC-MS/MS) analysis, after the in-gel digestion procedure as described by Della Corte and coll.[39] We list in table 1 the identified proteins with the correspondent NCBI accession number, the score, their isoelectric point (pI). Individual ions scores >36 indicate identity or extensive homology ($p<0.05$). Identified proteins include multiple form of yolk protein vitellogenin, heat shock protein (e.g., HSP8 and HSP70) and other proteins that have not been described before (indicated in table 1 with an asterisk).[40,41] These proteins are implicated in many pathways as in signalling, cell cycle regulation, protein trafficking, chaperoning, protein synthesis, and degradation.

TABLE 1. List of Proteins Identified Using the Nano Lc-Esi-Q-Tof in Zebrafish Embryo at Middle-Blastula-Gastrula Stage

With the Specification of Their NCBI Accession Number, Name, Score, Molecular Weight in Daltons, Isoelectric Point (pi) and Percentage Sequence Coverage.

Proteins highlighted with asterisk (*) had not so far been described in Zebrafish embryo.

Accession	Protein Name	Score	Molecular Weight	pI calculated	Sequence coverage
gi|166795887	vitellogenin 1 precursor	1108	150308	8,68	19
gi|94733730	vitellogenin 1	1039	149825	8,74	21
gi|94733733	novel protein similar to vitellogenin 1 (vg1)	913	149828	8,92	19
gi|94733734	novel protein similar to vitellogenin 1 (vg1)	835	150550	8,83	16
gi|145337918	Vtg1 protein	780	116965	9,07	18
gi|94733731	novel protein similar to vitellogenin 1 (vg1)	762	149911	8,84	19
gi|94732723	novel protein similar to vitellogenin 1 (vg1)	745	147826	8,73	17
gi|159155252*	Zgc:136383 protein	720	124413	8,78	17
gi|68448530	vitellogenin 5	559	149609	8,77	13
gi|92097636	Zgc:136383	402	28924	9,33	36
gi|63100501	Vtg1 protein	345	36580	9,23	28
gi|57864789	vitellogenin 7	341	24490	8,37	40
gi|57864783	vitellogenin 4	334	31304	9,48	27
gi|113678458	vitellogenin 2 isoform 1 precursor	323	181208	8,70	11
gi|125857991	Zgc:136383 protein	171	149328	8,93	9
gi|15209312*	procollagen type I alpha 2 chain	169	147826	9,35	4
gi|57864779	vitellogenin 2	122	69906	7,84	8
gi|11118642	vitellogenin 3 precursor	117	140477	6,92	2
gi|303227889	vitellogenin 6	73	151677	8,84	4
gi|13242157 *	egg envelope protein ZP2 variant A	71	48194	6,04	5
gi|6644111 *	nucleoside diphosphate kinase-Z1	69	17397	7,77	14
gi|18859071*	nucleoside diphosphate kinase 3	69	19558	7,68	7
gi|126632622*	novel prot. cont. a galactose binding lectin domain	67	19245	9,33	13
gi|66773080 *	mitochondrial ATP synthase beta subunit-like	66	55080	5,25	4
gi|38541767*	Ppia protein	60	19745	9,30	13
gi|1865782	HSC70 protein	58	71473	5,18	2
gi|28279108	heat shock protein 8	58	71382	5,32	4
gi|41152402*	histone H2B 3	49	13940	10,31	11
gi|41393113*	collagen, type I, alpha 1b precursor	46	137815	5,39	4
gi|94732492 *	ras homolog gene family, member F	46	24035	9,00	6
gi|47778620 *	tryptophan hydroxylase D2	45	55686	6,56	1
gi|68448517 *	zona pellucida glycoprotein 3.2 precursor	44	47365	4,92	2
gi|326677766 *	PREDICTED: RIMS-binding protein 2-like	41	138659	5,86	0
gi|112419298	Vtg3 protein	40	60622	6,32	2
gi|54400406 *	glutaredoxin 3	39	36541	5,18	11
gi|41152400*	peptidylprolyl isomerase A, like	37	17763	8,26	7

Ions score is $-10*Log(P)$, where P is the probability that the observed match is a random event.
Individual ions scores > 36 indicate identity or extensive homology (p<0.05).
Protein scores are derived from ions scores as a non-probabilistic basis for ranking protein hits.

Discussion and Conclusions

The use of stem cells differentiation factors in anticancer therapy has enabled one of us to build up a model of cancer corresponding to reality.[41] Such a model, conceived in 2002, describes cancer as a consequence of two different processes, i) a process of maturation arrest of stem cells (hierarchical model) and ii) a process of deterministic chaos in which genetic and epigenetic alterations conduce a normal differentiated cell to be malignant (stochastic model). In fact, these two processes are not mutually exclusive, and both have been described.[42,43]

Therefore, from this point of view, cancer cells can be defined as "cancer stem-like cells," that according to their degree of malignancy are considered blocked at a different phase of development. In fact, in tumors with an elevated degree of malignancy, such as acute lymphoblastic and myeloid leukemia, multipotent stem-like cells are present, whereas in tumors with lower malignancy, such as chronic lymphocytic leukemia, cells not yet completely differentiated are present, but toward a final differentiation.

In addition, cancer and stem cells share several characteristics. First, they present oncofetal antigens, maintained during the phylogenesis[44] and specific receptor on the cellular membrane on which the stem cells differentiation factors probably act. It has already been mentioned above that such factors could activate pathways of cellular differentiation that lead the cells to differentiate or to die, as usually occurs in the embryo (the apoptotic events in the embryo are many).

Furthermore, cancer and embryonic cells share common metabolic pathways such as APC/beta catenin/TCF/Wnt and the Hedgehog/Smoothened/Patched pathways.

The gene configuration and the metabolism of cancer cells is actually very similar to that of stem cells: they both have active proto-oncogene and produce embryonic growth factors, present oncofetal antigens, and work with an aerobic metabolism.

Nevertheless, cancer cells and stem cells show an important difference. The problem of cancer cells is double: they present genetic mutations that are at the origin of malignancy, and at the same time, they show an imbalance of the epigenetic code. In contrast with normal stem cells, tumor cells are not able to complete their development and to differentiate because they lost information; i.e., they experienced a mutation or epigenetic alterations in their code. The regulation of DNA information using epigenetic regulators such as SCDSFs, taken in the late stages of development of the embryo, transforms the cancer cells into normal cells or causes their apoptosis.

It is now emerging more and more clearly that the transcription factors, the microRNAs, the translational- and post-translational factors, play a fundamental role in the regulation of DNA information and in regulating the cell life. In other words, the epigenetic regulators contained in SCDSFs are able to differentiate and regulate normal stem cells and cancer stem cells, deactivating genes that lead cancer stem cells to proliferate while activating new differentiating pathways.

Our studies have recently been confirmed by other experimental researches performed by some colleagues of the Children's Hospital of Chicago.[12] In particular, they have confirmed that malignant melanoma reverts to a normal phenotype when it is in the environment of Zebrafish embryo. On the other hand there are many studies that highlight the link between tumor malignancy and the presence of cancer stem cells,[45] that seem to be resistant to conventional therapy, such as chemo- and radiotherapy. In the last 6–7 years scientific works in this field are so numerous that it is almost impossible to name all of them. Here we mention only those researches that demonstrated the presence of tumoral stem cell in breast cancer,[46,47,48,49,50,51] lung cancer,[52,53,53,55] prostate,[56,57,58] ovary cancer,[59,60,61,62,63] liver cancer,[64,65,66,67,68,69] stomach cancer,[70,71,72,73,74] colon cancer,[75,76,77] pancreas cancer,[78,79,80] glioblastoma multiforme,[81,82,83] head and neck cancer.[84,85,86,87] On the other hand, it is known that malignancy of many haematological tumoral diseases is due to the presence of stem cells.

Regarding the interpretation of the results obtained by using SCDSFs for the prevention of the neurodegenerative and for the treatment of psoriasis, we can assume that: the differentiation factors are epigenetic regulators, that on the one hand prevent the processes and the development of degenerative phenomena and on the other hand regulate the processes of abnormal cellular multiplication, as it comes, for instance, in psoriasis, where the multiplication of cells of the epithelial basal layer is five- to tenfold higher than that considered physiological. In this case we have demonstrated that the differentiation factors reduce the proliferation of the epidermal layers by normalizing it. In addition, other researches demonstrated that it is possible to tune in a fine way the fate of normal stem cells, like human mesenchymal stem cells, using SCDSFs. In fact, if we use in a specific way the different networks of substances present in the different stages of cell differentiation we can induce stem cells toward senescence or apoptosis (late stages of differentiation) or, at the contrary, enhance stem cell expression of multipotency by activating both telomerase-dependent and -independent antagonists of cell senescence (early stage of differentiation). Noteworthy, different modulating effects can be obtained only with a specific network of SCDSFs. From this point of view, the experiments about the prevention of neurodegeneration are enlightening. In fact, to prevent neurodegeneration, first of all we have to enhance stem-cell expression of multipotency, and then we have to induce stem cells toward differentiation in neural cells. For these reasons, all different stage factors expressed during cell differentiation have to be used: only the redundancy of these factors could lead to obtain significant results. These results lead us to consider a major shift in scientific paradigm (from reductionism to complexity) for preparing new treatments for chronic and degenerative diseases. In fact, these diseases entail an unexpected degree of complexity and disregulation, making the single-molecule-to-specific-target paradigm totally obsolete and inadequate. Rather, only a systemic approach can be envisioned as a successful strategy to deal with such complexity.

We believe that time is ready for a "metadisciplinary approach" in the treatment of degenerative diseases involving multiple tissues and organs, to help users in a new culture of collaboration from different scientific disciplines join together to combine their knowledge and come up with innovations, new therapeutic approaches, and most of all the development of novel paradigms. This is overdue to provide a reliable effort to help elderly people and everyone who suffers from degenerative diseases or cancer.

List of Abbreviations
Stem Cell Differentiation Stage Factors (SCDSFs), human Adipose-derived Stem Cells (hASCs), induced Pluripotent Stem cells (iPS), amino-acid (aa), Mitogen-Activated Protein Kinase (MAPK), Retinoblastoma protein (pRb), 5-Fluorouracil (5-Fu), human Colon cancer cells (Caco-2), N-Methyl-D-Aspartate (NMDA), Propidium Iodide (PI), Dulbecco Phosphate Buffered Saline (DPBS), hepato-cellular carcinoma (HCC), Hepatocyte Growth Factor (HGF), Fetal Calf Serum (FCS), Epidermal Growth Factor (EGF), Sodium Dodecyl Sulphate-PolyAcrylamide Gel Electrophoresis (SDS-PAGE), Liquid Chromatography–Mass Spectrometry (LC-MS/MS), Isoelectric point (pI), Heat Shock Protein (HSP).

References
1. Einhorn, L. Are there factors preventing cancer development during embryonic life? *Oncodev. Biol. Med.*, 1983, *4*(3), 219–229.
2. Lakshmi, M.S.; Sherbet, G.V. In: *Embryonic and Tumor Cell Interactions*; Sherbet G.V., Ed.; Karger Basel: New York, 1974; pp. 380–399.
3. Brent, R.L. Radiation Teratogenesis. *Teratology*, 1980, *21*(3), 281–298.
4. Pierce, G.B. The cancer cell and its control by the embryo. Rous-Whipple Award lecture. *Am. J. Pathol.*, 1983, *113*(1), 117–124.
5. Yu, C.L.; Tsai, M.H. Fetal fetuin selectively induces apoptosis in cancer cell lines and shows anti-cancer activity in tumor animal models. *Cancer Letter*, 2001, *166*(2), 173–184.
6. Papaioannou, V.E.; McBurney, M.V.; Gardner, R.L.; Evans, M.J. Fate of

teratocarcinoma cells injected into early mouse embryos. *Nature*, 1975, *258*(5530), 70–73.

7. Topczewska, J.M.; Postovit, L.M.; Margaryan, N.V.; Sam, A.; Hess, A.R.; Wheaton, W.W.; Nickoloff, B.J.; Topczewski, J.; Hendrix, M.J. Embryonic and tumorigenic pathways converge via Nodal signaling: role in melanoma aggressiveness. *Nat. Med.*, 2006, *12*(8), 925–932.

8. Kulesa, P.M.; Kasermeier-Kulesa, J.C.; Teddy, J.M.; Margaryan, N.V.; Seftor, E.A.; Seftor, R.E.; Hendrix, M.J. Reprogramming metastatic melanoma cells to assume a neural crest cell-like phenotype in an embryonic microenvironment. *Proc. Natl. Acad. Sci. USA*, 2006, *103*(10), 3752–3757.

9. Webb, C.G.; Gootwine, E.; Sachs, L. Developmental potential of myeloid leukemia cells injected into rat midgestation embryos. *Dev Biol.*, 1984, *101*(1), 221–224.

10. Weaver, V.M.; Petersen, O.W.; Wang, F.; Larabell, C.A.; Briand, P.; Damsky, C.; Bissell, M.J. Reversion of the malignant phenotype of human breast cells in three-dimensional culture and in vivo by integrin blocking antibodies. *J. Cell Biol.*, 1997, *137*(1), 231–245.

11. Coleman, W.B.; Wennerberg, A.E.; Smith, G.J.; Grisham, J.W. Regulation of the differentiation of diploid and some aneuploid rat liver epithelial (stem-like) cells by the hepatic microenvironment. *Am. J. Pathol.*, 1993, *142*(5), 1373–1382.

12. Postovit, L.M.; Maragaryan, N.V.; Seftor, E.A.; Kirschmann, D.A.; Lipavsky, A.; Wheaton, W.W.; Abbott, D.E.; Seftor, R.E.; Hendrix, M.J. Human embryonic stem cell microenvironment suppresses the tumorigenic phenotype of aggressive cancer cells. *Proc. Natl. Acad. Sci. USA,* 2008, *105*(11), 4329–4334.

13. Gallagher, J.M.; Komati, H.; Roy, E.; Nemer, M.; Latinkic, B.V. Dissociation of cardiogenic and postnatal myocardial activities of GATA4. *Mol. Cell Biol.*, 2012, *32*(12), 2214–2223.

14. Rizzi, R.; Di Pasquale, E.; Portararo, P.; Papait, R.; Cattaneo, P.; Latronico, M.V.; Altomare, C.; Sala, L.; Zaza, A.; Hirsch, E.; Naldini, L.; Condorelli, G.; Bearzi, C. Post-natal cardiomyocytes can generate iPS cells with an enhanced capacity toward cardiomyogenic re-differentiation. *Cell Death Differ.*, 2012, *19*(7), 1162–1174.

15. Ming, G.L.; Song, H. Adult neurogenesis in the mammalian brain: significant answers and significant questions. *Neuron*, 2011, *70*(4), 687–702.

16. Livraghi, T.; Meloni, F.; Frosi, A.; Lazzaroni, S.; Bizzarri, T.M.; Frati, L.; Biava, P.M. Treatment with stem cell differentiation stage factors of

intermediate-advanced hepatocellular carcinoma: an open randomized clinical trial. *Oncol. Res.*, 2005, *15* (7–8), 399–408.

17. Livraghi, T.; Ceriani, R.; Palmisano, A.; Pedicini, V.; Pich, M.G.; Tommasini, M.A.; Torzilli, G. Complete response in 5 out of 38 patients with advanced hepatocellular carcinoma treated with stem cell differentiation stage factors: case reports from a single centre. *Curr. Pharm. Biotechnol.*, 2011, *12*(2), 254–260.

18. Canaider, S.; Maioli, M.; Facchin, F.; Bianconi, E.; Santaniello, S.; Pigliaru, G.; Ljungberg, L.; Burigana, F; Bianchi, F.; Olivi, E.; Tremolada, C.; Biava, P.M.; Ventura, C. Human Stem Cell Exposure to Developmental Stage Zebrafish Extracts: a Novel Strategy for Tuning Stemness and Senescence Patterning. *CellR4*, 2014, *2*(5), e1226.

19. Di Pierro, F.; Negri, M.; Bollero, C. Terapia della psoriasi. Efficacia clinica di un preparato multicomponente. *Cosmetic Technology*, 2009, *12*(2), 13–17.

20. Harak, H.; Frosi, A.; Biava, P.M. Studio clinico sull'efficacia e tollerabilita' di una crema per uso topico nel trattamento della psoriasi. *La Med. Biol.*, 2012, *3*, 27–31.

21. Calzavara-Pinton, P.; Rossi, M. A topical remedy in association with phototherapy. Efficacy evaluation in patients suffering from moderate psoriasis. *Hi.tech dermo*, 2012, *1*, 41–47.

22. Plikus, M.V.; Van Spyk, E.N.; Pham, K.; Geyfman, M.; Kumar, V.; Takahashi, J.S.; Andersen, B. The Circadian Clock in Skin: Implications for Adult Stem Cells, Tissue Regeneration, Cancer, Aging, and Immunity. *J Biol. Rhythms.*, 2015, pii: 0748730414563537.

23. Hou, R.; Liu, R.; Niu, X.; Chang, W.; Yan, X.; Wang, C.; Li, J.; An, P.; Li, X.; Yin, G.; Zhang, K. Biological characteristics and gene expression pattern of bone marrow mesenchymal stem cells in patients with psoriasis. *Exp. Dermatol.*, 2014, *23*(7), 521–523.

24. Biava, P.M.; Bonsignorio, D.; Hoxa, M. Cell proliferation curves of different human tumor lines after in vitro treatment with Zebrafish embryonic extracts. *J. Tumor Marker Oncol.*, 2001, *16*(3), 195–202.

25. Biava, P.M.; Carluccio, A. Activation of anti-oncogene p53 produced by embryonic extracts in vitro tumor cells. *J. Tumor Marker Oncol.*, 1977, *12*(4), 9–15.

26. Biava, P.M.; Bonsignorio, D.; Hoxa, M.; Impagliazzo, M.; Facco, R.; Ielapi, T.; Frati, L.; Bizzarri, M. Post-translational modification of the retinoblastoma protein (pRb) induced by in vitro administration of Zebrafish embryonic extracts on human kidney adenocarcinoma cell line. *J. Tumor Marker Oncol.*, 2002, *17*(2), 59–64.

27. Cucina, A.; Biava, P.M.; D'Anselmi, F.; Coluccia, P.; Conti, F.; di Clemente, R.; Miccheli, A.; Frati, L.; Gulino, A.; Bizzarri, M. Zebrafish embryo proteins induce apoptosis in human colon cancer cells (Caco2). *Apoptosis*, 2006, *11*(9), 1617–1628.

28. D'Anselmi, F.; Cucina, A.; Biava, P.M.; Proietti, S.; Coluccia, P.; Frati, L.; Bizzarri, M. Zebrafish stem cell differentiation stage factors suppress Bcl-xL release and enhance 5-Fu-mediated apoptosis in colon cancer cells. *Curr. Pharm. Biotechnol.*, 2011, *12*(2), 261–267.

29. Biava, P.M.; Nicolini, A.; Ferrari, P.; Carpi, A.; Sell, S. A systemic approach to cancer treatment: tumor cell reprogramming focused on endocrine-related cancers. *Curr. Med. Chem.*, 2014, *21*(9), 1072–1081.

30. Bianchi, F.; Maioli, M.; Leonardi, E.; Olivi, E.; Pasquinelli, G.; Valente, S.; Mendez, A.J.; Ricordi, C.; Raffaini, M.; Tremolada, C.; Ventura, C. A new non enzymatic method and device to obtain a fat tissue derivative highly enriched in pericyte-like elements by mild mechanical forces from human lipoaspirates. *Cell Transplant.*, 2013, *22*(11), 2063–2077.

31. Conner, E.A.; Teramoto, T.; Wirth, P.J.; Kiss, A.; Garfield, S.; Thorgeirsson, S.S. HGF-mediated apoptosis via p53/bax-independent pathway activating JNK1. *Carcinogenesis*, 1999, *20*(4), 583–590.

32. Feng, R.; Zhou, S.; Liu, Y.; Song, D.; Luan, Z.; Dai, X.; Li, Y.; Tang, N.; Wen, J.; Li, L. Sox2 protects neural stem cells from apoptosis via up regulating survivin expression. *Biochem. J.*, 2013, *450*(3), 459–468.

33. Park, I.K.; Qian, D.; Kiel, M.; Becker, M.W.; Pihalja, M.; Weissman, I.L.; Morrison, S.J.; Clarke, M.F. Bmi-1 is required for maintenance of adult self-renewing hematopioetic stem cells. *Nature*, 2003, *423*(6937), 302–305.

34. Gardoni, F.; Bellone, C.; Viviani, B.; Marinovich, M.; Meli, E.; Pellegrini-Giampietro, D.E.; Cattabeni, F.; Di Luca, M. Lack of PSD-95 drives hippocampal neuronal cell death through activation of an alpha CaMKII transduction pathway. *Eur. J. Neurosci.*, 2002, *16*(5), 777–786.

35. Pellegrini-Giampietro, D.E.; Cozzi, A.; Peruginelli, F.; Leonardi, P.; Meli, E.; Pellicciari, R.; Moroni, F. 1-Aminoindan-1,5-dicarboxylic acid and (S)-(+)-2-(3'-carboxybicyclo [1.1.1] pentyl)-glycine, two mGlu1 receptor-preferring antagonists, reduce neuronal death in in vitro and in vivo models of cerebral ischaemia. *Eur. J. Neurosci.*, 1999, *11*(10), 3637–3647.

36. Norata, G.D.; Biava, P.M.; Di Pierro, F. The Zebrafish embryo derivative affects cell viability of epidermal cells: a possible role in the treatment of psoriasis. *G. Ital. Dermatol. Venereol.*, 2013, *148*(5), 479–483.

37. Shi, Q.; Jackowski, G. In: *Gel Electrophoresis of Proteins: A Practical Approach*, 3rd ed.; Hames, Ed.; Oxford University Press Inc: New York, 1998; Chap. 1, 13–29.

38. Kang, D.H.; Gho, Y.S.; Suh, M.K.; Kang, C.H. Highly sensitive and fast protein detection with coomassie brilliant blue in sodium dodecyl sulfate-polyacrylamide gel electrophoresis. *Bull. Korean Chem. Soc.*, 2002, *23*, 1511–1512.

39. Della Corte, A.; Tamburrelli, C.; Crescente, M.; Giordano, L.; D'Imperio, M.; Di Michele, M.; Donati, M.B.; De Gaetano, G.; Rotilio, D.; Cerletti, C. Platelet proteome in healthy volunteers who smoke. *Platelets*, 2012, *23*(2), 91–105.

40. Lucitt, M.B.; Price, T.S.; Pizarro, A.; Wu, W.; Yocum, A.K.; Seiler, C.; Pack, M.A.; Blair, I.A.; Fitzgerald, G.A.; Grosser T. Analysis of the Zebrafish proteome during embryonic development. *Mol. Cell. Proteomics*, 2008, *7*(5), 981–994.

41. Biava, P.M.; Bonsignorio, D. Cancer and cell differentiation: a model to explain malignancy. *J. Tumor Marker Oncol.*, 2002, *17*(2), 47–54.

42. Shackleton, M.; Quintana, E.; Fearon, E.R.; Morrison, S.J. Heterogeneity in cancer: cancer stem cells versus clonal evolution. *Cell*, 2009, *138*(5), 822–829.

43. Visvader, J.E.; Lindeman, G.J. Cancer stem cells: current status and evolving complexities. *Cell Stem Cell.*, 2012, *10*(6), 717–728.

44. Biava, P.M; Monguzzi, A; Bonsignorio, D; Frosi, A; Sell, S; Klavins, J.V. Xenopus laevis Embryos share antigens with Zebrafish Embryos and with human malignant neoplasms. *J. Tumor Marker Oncol.*, 2001, *16*(3), 203–206.

45. Reya, T.; Morrison, S.J.; Clarke, M.F.; Weissman, I.L. Stem cells, cancer and cancer stem cells. *Nature*, 2001, *414*(6859), 105–111.

46. Chen, J.; Chen, Z.L. Technology update for the sorting and identification of breast cancer stem cells. *Chin. J. Cancer*, 2010, *29*(3), 265–269.

47. Roesler, R.; Cornelio, D.B.; Abujamra, A.L.; Schwartsmann, G. HER2 as a cancer stem-cell target. *Lancet Oncol.*, 2010, *11*(3), 225–226.

48. Wu, W. Patents related to cancer stem cell research. *Recent Pat. DNA Gene Seq.*, 2010, *4*(1), 40–45.

49. Park, S.Y.; Lee, H.E.; Li, H.; Shipitsin, M.; Gelman, R.; Polyak, K. Heterogeneity for stem cell-related markers according to tumor subtype and histologic stage in breast cancer. *Clin. Cancer Res.*, 2010, *16*(3), 876–887.

50. Lawson, J.C.; Blatch, G.L.; Edkins, A.L. Cancer stem cells in breast cancer and metastasis. *Breast Cancer Res. Treat.*, 2009, *118*(2), 241–254.

51. Luo, J.; Yin, X.; Ma, T.; Lu, J. Stem cells in normal mammary gland and breast cancer. *Am. J. Med. Sci.*, 2010, *339*(4), 366–370.

52. Spiro, S.G.; Tanner, N.T.; Silvestri, G.A.; Janes, S.M.; Lim, E.; Vansteenkiste, J.F.; Pirker, R. Lung cancer: progress in diagnosis staging and therapy. *Respirology*, 2010, *15*(1), 44–50.

53. Gorelik, E.; Lokshin, A.; Levina, V. Lung cancer stem cells as a target for therapy. *Anticancer Agents Med. Chem.*, 2010, *10*(2), 164–171.

54. Sullivan, J.P.; Minna, J.D.; Shay, J.W. Evidence for self-renewing lung cancer stem cells and their implications in tumor initiation, progression and targeted therapy. *Cancer Metastasis Rev.*, 2010, *29*(1), 61–72.

55. Westhoff, B.; Colaluca, I.N.; D'Ario, G.; Donzelli, M.; Tosoni, D.; Volorio, S.; Pelosi, G.; Spaggiari, L.; Mazzarol, G.; Viale, G.; Pece, S.; Di Fiore, P.P. Alterations of the Notch pathway in lung cancer. *Proc. Natl. Acad. Sci. USA*, 2009, *106*(52), 22293–22298.

56. Lawson, D.A.; Zong, Y.; Memarzadeh, S.; Xin, L.; Huang, J.; Witte, O.N. Basal epithelial stem cells are efficient targets for prostate cancer initiation. *Proc. Natl. Acad. Sci. USA*, 2010, *107*(6), 2610–2615.

57. Lang, S.H.; Anderson, E.; Fordham, R.; Collins, A.T. Modeling the prostate stem cell niche: an evaluation of stem cell survival and expansion in vitro. *Stem. Cells Dev.*, 2010, *19*(4), 537–546.

58. Joung, J. Y.; Cho, K. S.; Kim, J. E.; Seo, H.K.; Chung, J.; Park, W. S.; Choi, M.K.; Lee, K.H. Prostate stem cell antigen mRNA in peripheral blood as a potential predictor of biochemical recurrence of metastatic prostate cancer. *J. Surg. Oncol.*, 2010, *101*(2), 145–148.

59. Liu, T.; Cheng, W.; Lai, D.; Huang, Y.; Guo, L. Characterization of primary ovarian cancer cells in different culture systems. *Oncol. Rep.*, 2010, *23*(5), 1277–1284.

60. Fong, M.Y.; Kakar, S.S. The role of cancer stem cells and the side population in epithelial ovarian cancer. *Histol. Histopathol.*, 2010, *25*(1), 113–120.

61. Murphy, S.K. Targeting ovarian cancer-initiating cells. *Anticancer Agents Med. Chem.*, 2010, *10*(2), 157–163.

62. Peng, S.; Maihle, N.J.; Huang, Y. Pluripotency factors Lin 28 and Oct 4 identify a sub-population of stem cell-like cells in ovarian cancer. *Oncogene*, 2010, *29*(14), 2153–2159.

63. Kusumbe, A. P.; Bapat, S. A. Cancer stem cells and aneuploid populations within developing tumors are the major determinants of tumor dormancy. *Cancer Res.*, 2009, *69*(24), 9245–9253.

64. Tomuleasa, C.; Soritau, O.; Rus-Ciuca, D.; Pop, T.; Todea, D.; Mosteanu, O.; Pintea, B.; Foris, V.; Susman, S.; Kacso, G.; Irimie, A. Isolation and characterization of hepatic cells with stem-like properties from hepatocellular carcinoma. *J. Gastrointestin. Liver Dis.*, 2010, *19*(1), 61–67.

65. Zou, G.M. Liver cancer stem cells as an important target in liver cancer therapies. *Anticancer Agents Med. Chem.*, 2010, *10*(2), 172–175.

66. Lee, T.K.; Castilho, A.; Ma, S.; Ng, I.O. Liver cancer stem cells: implications for new therapeutic target. *Liver Int.*, 2009, *29*(7), 955–965.

67. Marquardt, J.U.; Thorgeirsson, S.S. Stem Cells in hepatocarcinogenesis: evidence from genomic data. *Semin. Liver Dis.*, 2010, *30*(1), 26–34.

68. Kung, J.W.; Currie, I. S.; Forbes, S. J.; Ross, J. A. Liver development, regeneration, and carcinogenesis. *J. Biomed. Biotechnol.*, 2010, *2010*, 984248.

69. Gai, H.; Nguyen, D.M.; Moon, Y.J.; Aguila, J.R.; Fink, L.M.; Ward, D.C.; Ma, Y. Generation of murine hepatic lineage cells from induced pluripotent stem cells. *Differentiation*, 2010, *79*(3), 171–181.

70. Correia, M.; Machado, J.C.; Ristimaki, A. Basic aspects of gastric cancer. *Helicobacter*, 2009, *14*(1), 36–40.

71. Takaishi, S.; Okumura,T.; Tu, S.; Wang, S.S.; Shibata, W.; Vigneshwaran, R.; Gordon, S.A.; Shimada, Y.; Wang, T.C. Identification of gastric cancer stem cells using the surface marker CD44. *Stem Cells*, 2009, *27*(5), 1006–1020.

72. Nishii, T.; Yashiro, M.; Shinto, O.; Sawada, T.; Ohira, M.; Hirakawa, K. Cancer stem cell-like SP cells have a high adhesion ability to the peritoneum in gastric carcinoma. *Cancer Sci.*, 2009, *100*(8), 1397–1402.

73. Chen, Z.; Xu, W. R.; Qian, H.; Zhu, W.; Bu, X.F.; Wang, S.; Yan, Y.M.; Mao, F.; Gu, H. B.; Cao, H. L.; Xu, X. J. Oct4, a novel marker for human gastric cancer. *J. Surg. Oncol.*, 2009, *99*(7), 414–419.

74. Kang, D.H.; Han, M.E.; Song, M.H.; Lee, Y.S.; Kim, E.H.; Kim, H.J.; Kim, G.H.; Kim, D.H.; Yoon, S.; Baek, S.Y.; Kim, B.S.; Kim, J.B.; Oh, S.O. The role of hedgehog signaling during gastric regeneration. *J. Gastroenterol.*, 2009, *44*(5), 372–379.

75. Yeung, T.M.; Ghandhi, S.C.; Wilding, J.L.; Muschel, R.; Bodmer, W.F. Cancer stem cells from colorectal cancer derived cell lines. *Proc. Natl. Acad. Sci. USA*, 2010, *107*(8), 3722–3727.

76. Gulino, A.; Ferretti, E.; De Smaele, E. Hedgehog signaling in colon cancer and stem cells. *EMBO Mol. Med.*, 2009, *1*(6–7), 300–302.

77. Thenappan, A.; Li, Y.; Shetty, K.; Johnson, L.; Reddy, E.P.; Mishra, L. New

therapeutic targeting colon cancer stem cells. *Curr. Colorectal Cancer Rep.*, 2009, *5*(4), 209.

78. Rasheed, Z.A.; Yang, J.; Wang, Q.; Kowalski, J.; Freed, I.; Murter, C.; Hong, S. M.; Koorstra, J.B.; Rajeshkumar, N. V.; He, X.; Goggins, M.; Iacobuzio-Donahue, C.; Berman, D. M.; Laheru, D.; Jimeno, A.; Hidalgo, M.; Maitra, A.; Matsui, W. Prognostic significance of tumorigenic cells with mesenchymal features in pancreatic adenocarcinoma. *J. Natl. Cancer Inst.*, 2010, *102*(5), 340–351.

79. Puri, S.; Hebrok, M. Cellular plasticity within pancreas—lessons learned from development. *Dev. Cell*, 2010, *18*(3), 342–356.

80. Quante, M.; Wang, T. C. Stem cells in gastroenterology and hepatology. *Nat. Rev. Gastroenterol. Hepatol.*, 2009, *6*(12), 724–737.

81. Sato, A.; Sakurada, K.; Kumabe, T.; Sasajima, T.; Beppu, T.; Asano, K.; Ohkuma, H.; Ogawa, A.; Mizoi, K.; Tominaga, T.; Kitanaka, C.; Kayama, T.; Tohoku Brain Tumor Study Group. Association of stem cell marker CD133 expression with dissemination of glioblastoma. *Neurosurg. Rev.*, 2010, *33*(2), 175–183.

82. Di Tomaso, T.; Mazzoleni, S.; Wang, E.; Sovena, G.; Clavenna, D.; Franzin, A.; Mortini, P.; Ferrone, S.; Doglioni, C.; Marincola, F. M.; Galli, R.; Parmiani, G.; Maccalli, C. Immunobiological characterization of cancer stem cells isolated from glioblastoma patients. *Clin. Cancer Res.*, 2010, *16*(3), 800–813.

83. Ji, J.; Black, K.L.; Yu, J.S. Glioma stem cell research for the development of immunotherapy. *Neurosurg. Clin. N. Am.*, 2010, *21*(1), 159–166.

84. Ailles, L.; Prince, M. Cancer stem cells in head and neck squamous cell carcinoma. *Methods Mol. Biol.*, 2009, *568*, 175–193.

85. Zhang, P.; Zhang, Y.; Mao, L.; Zhang, Z.; Chen, W. Side population in oral squamous cell carcinoma possesses tumor stem cell phenotype. *Cancer Lett.*, 2009, *277*(2), 227–234.

86. Brunner M.; Thurnher, D.; Heiduschka, G.; Grasl, M.Ch.; Brostjan, C.; Erovic, B. M. Elevated levels of circulating endothelial progenitor cells in head and neck cancer patients. *J. Surg. Oncol.*, 2008, *98*(7), 545–550.

87. Zhang, Q.; Shi, S.; Yen, Y.; Brown, J.; Ta, J.Q.; Le, A.D. A subpopulation of CD133(+) cancer stem-like cells characterized in human oral squamous cell carcinoma confer resistance to chemotherapy. *Cancer Lett.*, 2010, *289*(2), 151–160.

Getting an Insight into the Complexity of Major Chronic Inflammatory and Degenerative Diseases: A Possible New Systemic Approach to Their Treatment

Current Pharmaceutical Biotechnology, 2015, Volume 16, Number 9: 793–803. © Bentham Science Publishers.

P. M. Biava, G. Norbiato

This paper describes why chronic diseases, including not only cancer, but also the metabolic syndrome, chronic inflammation, chronic degenerative diseases, and others, make diagnosis, prevention, and targeted therapeutic treatment particularly difficult. Recognition that chronic inflammation may induce genetic, neuro-endocrine, immune, and metabolic changes in a series of diseases can be used for designing new approaches to treatment. This study suggests a new approach, including reprogramming. The use of stem cell differentiation stage factors as epigenetic reprogramming factors of all cells of the psycho-neuro-endocrine-immune system can restore the balance of a system that has been disrupted by chronic inflammation.

Introduction

Exposure to threats to body homeostasis promotes survival through activation of multiple interacting systems including the behavioral, neuro-endocrine, immune, and metabolic systems that produce an integrated stress response. While the response is initially adaptive, prolonged activation of these systems becomes maladaptive by inducing pronounced changes in body physiology and behavior that have deleterious implications for survival and well-being. The immune system is recognized best for its role in protection against pathogens that cause disease. However, immune activation is not solely relegated to attack against foreign pathogens, but plays an integral role regulating homeostatic conditions related to immune surveillance against tumor genesis and chronic inflammatory diseases. Thus the immune system represents a complex network requiring tight regulatory control and the interaction between neuro-endocrine and immune system is believed to be essential in defining the mechanism regulating infectious and non-infectious disease states.[1-2] It is now accepted that the nervous system can receive input from the immune system via the release of cytokines and other immune mediators.[3] At the same time, the immune system is also receptive to signals conveyed from neuro-endocrine and neuro-transmitter-mediated signals suggesting a bi-directional interplay between the release of neuro-endocrine hormone factors and cytokines.[4-5] The integration of metabolism and immunity can be traced back to an evolutionary need for survival. Accordingly, the primary role of physiological adaptation is to find the energetically most efficient system configuration. In this sense a disease indicates a system-wide deterioration with declining efficiency of energy capture and utilization. The initiation and maintenance of immunity is a metabolically costly process. Sepsis can increase human metabolic rate by 30–60% and maintenance of phagocytes during infection needs approximately the same energy consumption.[6] Inflammation, glucocorticoids, and insulin signaling pathways also proved to be involved in metabolic physiological adaptation linked programs.

Glucocorticoids (GCs) are essential endocrine hormones, involved in the regulation of almost all major physiological functions, including energy metabolism, cell proliferation and differentiation, reproduction, immune system, and cardiovascular and brain function. Further GCs, which are with insulin the main metabolic hormones, have an important metabolic function as they provide substrates for oxidative metabolism by increasing hepatic glucose production, adipose tissues lipolysis, and proteolysis. Binding insulin to its receptor triggers the tyrosine phosphorylation of its cellular substrate, such as the insulin receptor substrate family protein[7] that is crucial signaling and molecular events for many metabolic effects of insulin.[7,8] Insulin effects are inhibited during stress and inflammation through modification of serine phosphorylation, mediated by intracellular pathways. Modifications that impair action from insulin can be triggered by increased cortisol activity, pro-inflammatory cytokines, and nutrients such as lipids.[8] Inhibitory effects of inflammation on peripheral insulin sensitivity have been observed in obesity, in subjects suffering from insulin resistance and type-2 diabetes. GCs play a major role in the body response to stress and inflammation, maintaining a complex tightly balanced system in the brain and periphery that translates the effect of stress on specific tissues. Stress and inflammation are potential factors for a large number of diseases, ranging from peripheral illness such as diabetes, obesity, cardiovascular diseases, cancer,[9,10,11] to many psychiatric disorders,[12] including major depression, schizophrenia, drug addiction, post-traumatic stress disorder, and Alzheimer's disease.[13]

The prevalence of these diseases has increased rapidly over the past decades. A great proportion of global disorders involves the failure to resolve inflammation that appears to be chronic from the onset. However, acute and chronic inflammation may coexist over long periods implying continuous re-initiation. Post-inflammatory tissue repair requires the coordinate restitution of different cell type and structures including epithelium, mesenchymal cells, extracellular matrix, and vasculature. So, inappropriate reconstruction of inflammatory tissues may preclude repair, resulting in atrophy, fibrosis, and damages to tissue function, which in turn activates inflammation.

Since inflammatory mechanisms are dominant over homeostatic control, thus inflammatory mediators may alter the homeostatic control leading to alterations of a complex regulatory network in which different adaptive systems, such as the neuro-endocrine-immune-metabolic systems, work continuously in concert establishing new equilibria. This characteristic accounts for the pathological strength of chronic inflammatory responses.[9]

Energy regulation (EnR) is the most important factor for homeostatic regulation of physiological processes. Neuro-endocrine pathways are involved in EnR. Insulin, insulin-like growth factor, estrogen, androgen, and hosteocalcin are factors that provide energy-rich fuels to stores, while hypothalamic pituitary adrenal axis, the sympathetic system, thyroid hormones, glucagon, and growth hormones provide energy-rich substrate to consumers. It is hypothesized that unresolved inflammation involves the entire body to divert fuels to the activated immune system. As EnR and the neuro-endocrine-immune interplay have not evolved to cope with long-lasting chronic inflammation, the coordination of the interlinked pathways will not function in chronic inflammation as expected for short-lasting diseases. The abnormal control leads to multiple disease-related sequelae, the pathogenesis of which can be explained by alteration of EnR and, subsequently, changes in the neuro-endocrine-immune-metabolic pathways. Physiopathology of energy regulation has been extensively reviewed.[14] The biologic complexity of unresolved inflammation and a limited understanding of dysfunctions underlying many chronic diseases, including the metabolic syndrome, brain diseases, and cancer, combine to make the diagnosis, prevention, and targeted therapeutic treatment particularly difficult. Moreover, every anti-inflammatory therapy now in use has one or more serious toxicity potentials, and medical treatments have not focused on pathogenic factors other than inflammation, the regulatory cure of noninfectious infection-associated diseases.[15] Recognition that chronic inflammation may induce epigenetic, genetic, neuro-endocrine, immune, and metabolic changes in a series of diseases is useful for designing new targets for prevention and treatment.[16]

The current review describes how unresolved inflammation plays an important role in high morbidity diseases including cancer, brain diseases, obesity, and HIV infection. Principal mediators, signaling pathways, biomarkers, and potential therapeutic implications are to be taken into consideration. Owing to the complexity of the networks involved in such diseases, a landscape analysis of inflammatory, immune, endocrine, metabolic, and oncogenic pathophenotypes has been performed, and biological treatment with stem cells differentiation stage factors has been proposed.

Cancer-Related Inflammation

It has long been recognized that the immune system plays a role in the development of tumors. Immune cells can suppress tumor development by killing tumor cells; conversely they can also promote tumor progression. A tumor can be completely eliminated or kept dormant by tumor inhibiting inflammation consisting in production of tumor inhibiting cytokines, in the infiltration of cells of both the innate immune system such as dendritic cells, natural killer cells, and the adaptive system TH1—CD4+ and CD8+.[17,18] In the escape phase a tumor often develops multiple mechanisms to evade anti-tumor cells-mediated destruction[19] and induction of immune suppressive micro-environment by tumor and stromal cells that promote cancer cells' proliferation and migration.[20] Approximately 18% of cancer cases worldwide are attributable to infectious diseases caused by bacteria, virus, and parasites, while inflammation can account for approximately 25–50% of human cancer. Key regulators of tumor progression are transcription factors, cytokines, reactive oxygen, nitrogen species (RONs), and gonadal hormones.

As can be seen, the collective immune effects of cytokines, micro RNA and RONs may be either pro- or anti-inflammatory or pro- and anti-tumorigenic, depending on their balance, thus increasing the complexity of the systems involved. The pathophysiology of cancer related inflammation has been extensively reviewed by Mantovani[21] and Schetter.[22]

Reactive Oxygen and Nitrogen Species (RONs)

An inflammatory stimulus leads to the recruitment and activation of various immune cells, including macrophages, neutrofils, and dendritic cells, that release reactive oxygen species and reactive nitrogen species (RONs). These radicals have a role for an efficient immune response that may be either tumorigenic or anti-tumorigenic depending on concentrations.[23] Increased RONs may cause genomic instability that contributes to carcinogenesis by mutating proto-oncogenes and tumor suppressor genes. Elevated RONs can post-translationary modify proteins, rendering them auto-antigenic, so increasing angiogenesis and metastatic potential. Parasites, viruses, helicobacter pilory are important risk factors for cholangiocarcinoma, epatocellular carcinoma, cervical and gastric cancer. RONs can be induced by various factors, including inflammatory cytokines and NFkB, hypoxia, and microbial endotoxin.[24] Whether nitric oxide (NO) produced by RONs has pro-tumorigenic and anti-tumorigenic effects depends on the status of p53 tumor suppressor gene, which, if activated, leads to growth arrest, DNA repair, apoptosis, and anti-carcinogenic effect. In the absence of functional p53 an inflammatory stimulus can lead to overproduction of (NO) leading to a tumorigenic condition.

Cytokines

Cytokines are signaling molecules that are key mediators of inflammation or immune response. Pro-inflammatory cytokines include IL-1, IL-6, IL-15, IL-17, IL-23, TNFα, and anti-inflammatory cytokines include IL-4, IL-10, IL-13, transforming growth factor, TGFß and interferon (INFα). Depending on the balance of cytokines, their collective effects may be either pro- or anti-inflammatory. Cytokines binding to membrane receptors activate signal transduction pathways that regulate apoptosis, cell proliferation, angiogenesis, and cellular senescence.[25] For example: TNFα, by activating the inflammation transcription factor NF-kB can increase tumor growth and the metastatic potential. IL-6 activates the Janus kinase signal transducer and other activators of transcriptor signal pathway that are tumorigenic.[26] IL-10 and TGFß are anti-inflammatory cytokines. The main function of IL-10 is to suppress NF-kB which is associated with inhibition of TNFα, IL-6 and IL-12.[27]

Along with NF-kB, STAT3 and IL-6 are a point of convergence of numerous oncogenic signal pathways.[26] The pro-inflammatory cytokines IL-1ß secreted by malignant cells of infiltrating leucocytes increases tumor adhesion and invasion, angiogenesis, and immune suppression.

Micro RNA

Micro RNAs are small, non-coding RNAs that regulate the translation of specific genes in inflammatory and cancer diseases. Stimuli that induce micro RNA expression include direct transcriptional activation or repression from transcriptional enhancers, epigenetic modification of the genome, genomic amplification or dilation, cellular stress, and inflammatory stimuli. Induction or repression of micro RNA expression influences cell fate, cell proliferation, DNA repair, DNA methylation, and apoptosis and provide pro-inflammatory or anti-inflammatory stimuli. Micro RNAs have an essential role in both adaptive and innate immune systems.[28]

Chronic Inflammation in the Tumor Micro-Environment

Key features of cancer related inflammation (CRI) include the infiltration of a wide number of blood cells, preeminently tumor-associated macrophages (TAMs); the presence of cytokines such as TNFα, IL-1, IL-6; chemokines such as CCL2 and CXCL8; and transcription factors.[29-30] Endogenous promoter NF-kB has a key role in regulating innate immunity both in tumors and inflammatory cells. Besides neoplastic cells, a tumor is composed of stroma containing fibroblast, vessels, and leucocytes. Pro-inflammatory cytokines TNF can involve enhanced tumor growth, invasion and inhibition of glucogen synthase kinase 3 Beta, that contribute to tumor development.[31-32] The pro-inflammatory cytokine IL-1 Beta, TNalfa, and IL6 are known to stimulate cancer cells to metastasize. IL-1 beta secreted by malignant cells or infiltrating leucocytes increases tumor adhesion and invasion, angiogenesis, and immune suppression. TAMs are principle leucocytes subset driving an amplification of the inflammatory response in the tumor.

Sex Steroid Hormones and Cancer

BREAST CANCER

Breast cancer continues to be the most common cancer in women and represents a major issue of public health.[33] The majority of estrogen receptors negative (ER-) breast cancers develop resistance to adjuvant hormone therapy and triple negative breast cancer lacks effective targeted treatment. Initially, tumors can be completely eliminated or kept in a dormant state by tumor-inhibiting inflammation characterized by the production of tumor-inhibiting cytokines and infiltration of cells of both the innate immune system such as dendrites cells (DCs) and natural killer (NK) cells and the adaptive immune system such as TH1, CD4+, and CD8+ T-cells.[34-35-36] In the escape phase, breast tumors may develop multiple mechanisms to evade immune surveillance that include the creation of autonomous cancer cells to evade anti-tumor cells, cell-mediated destruction, and the induction of an immunosuppressive microenvironment by tumor and/or stroma cells that directly promotes cancer cell proliferation and migration.[37] Immune cells can suppress tumor development or inhibit their growth; conversely they can promote tumor progression, establishing an immune suppressive micro-environment.

Biomarkers of breast cancer risks are: insulin resistance, estrogen resistance, hyperinsulinemia, and low grade chronic inflammation, which are major predictors of adiposity, diabetes risks, and breast cancer risks. Both non-tumoral and malignant breast tissue and cells are endowed with key enzymes of steroid metabolism, including 17beta hydroxysteroid dehydrogenase, 5beta-reductase and aromatase. Locally produced or metabolically transformed estrogen may differently affect proliferal activity of breast cancer cells.[38] Studies on breast cancer demonstrate that immune network and locally produced estrogens may play a significant role in the development and progression of breast cancer.

Altered insulin receptor binding promotes mitosis and anti-apoptotic effects in breast cancer cells and also tumor cell migration and tumor-associated angiogenesis. Chronically elevated insulin can enhance estrogen bio-activity and promote activities of breast cancer related adipokines.[39] Increased systemic reactive oxygen species (ROS) is hypothesized to play a central role in breast carcinogenesis and in carcinogenesis causal pathways linked to obesity.[40] Because telomeres (nucleoprotein repeats at the end of chromosomes that protect cells from chromosome instability) suffer disproportionately from oxidative damage, telomere attrition may be considered an important cause of breast cancer. Finally, global DNA hypo-methylation is recognized to be a key epigenetic mechanism associated with increased cancer risks, namely breast cancer risk.[41]

PROSTATE CANCER

Prostate cancer (PC) remains one of the most widespread cancers in males. The androgen receptor is the most regulatory transcription factor in cells of prostatic lineage, and this regulatory function is maintained in PC cells. The frontline treatment involves androgen deprivation therapy, which is achieved by blocking androgen production with surgery or androgen antagonist. Suppression of androgens/androgen receptors signaling is effective at improving cancer symptoms and prolonging survival. However, testosterone deficiency leads to the development of the metabolic syndrome suggesting that steps be taken early to manage metabolic complications associated with prostate cancer.[42] PC and inflammation are closely linked, so much that cancer patients show both local and systemic changes in inflammatory parameters.

In some cancer types, inflammatory conditions occur before malignant changes, whereas in different types of cancer, an oncogenic alteration generates an inflammatory micro-environment that induces development of tumors.[43] Recent studies uncovered the relation among estrogens and androgens, steroid hormones, cytokines IL-1 and IL-2, and prostate cancer. Androgen aromatization to estrogen may play a role in prostate carcinogenesis and tumor progression. Estrogens combined with androgens appear to be required for the malignant transformation of prostate epithelial cells.[44] Interestingly, IL-2 produced by macrophages in the tumor micro-environment converts androgen receptor from inhibitor to modulator, thus inducing resistance to hormonal therapies.[45]

The Brain and the Adaptive Stress System

The perception of a potential threatening situation activates the HPA axis, the paraventricular nucleus of the hypothalamus where corticotrophin-releasing hormone (CRH) and vasopressin stimulate ACTH, which in turn stimulates the adrenal glands to release cortisol in humans. Cortisol is a pleiotropic hormone that is involved in almost every cellular, molecular, and physiological phenotype essential for life. During evolution, several mechanisms appeared to allow a fine-tuned regulation of glucocorticoid signaling that includes glucocorticoid receptors (GRs), mineral corticoid receptors (MRs), and two enzymes, 11Beta hydroxy steroid dehydrogenase type-1 (11beta HSD-1) and type-2 (11Beta HSD-2) that interconvert active cortisol into inactive cortisone. The glucocorticoid receptors have a number of complex interactions with the epigenome. Epigenetic mechanisms are considered essential for the transduction of environmental inputs, like stress, into lasting physiological and behavioral changes. Stress has a number of effects on brain epigenetic mechanisms producing alterations in DNA methylation and histone modifications in most of the stress-sensitive brain regions.[46,47] Many of these changes may be maladaptive and contribute to neuro-degenerative and neuro-psychiatric diseases.

The GR is a ligand-regulated transcription factor member of the nuclear receptor superfamily, which controls gene expression linked to several processes like inflammation, stress response, glucose homeostasis, lipid metabolism, proliferation, and apoptosis development.[48] The biological action of glucocorticoids is mediated by intra-cellular GRs that, when bound to homologous ligand, function as DNA-bind protein that enhances or represses basal transcription rate of responsive genes. In most cells GCs promote reduction in GR levels and consequently limit the span of cellular responsiveness to GCs.[48] GCs act as the critical negative feedback on all myeloid cells, including those present within the brain parenchyma. An inappropriate feedback of GCs on microglia and high circulating GCs levels in stressed individuals have been associated with deleterious consequences for the brain.

Previous studies have proven involvement of G-protein and the signal regulated kinase-CREB pathway in rapid GCs effects.[49] This same pathway is also activated by rapid signaling of other steroid receptors, such as oestrogen, androgen, and progesterone receptors and by rapid aldosterone signaling through the MRs in peripheral tissues.[50] This suggests that a specific type of G-protein is engaged in multiple hormone actions in the brain and periphery and gives reason of glucocorticoids, mineralocorticoids, and sex hormones involvement in chronic inflammatory diseases and correlated disorders. Gonadal steroids have a similar capacity to produce epigenomic reorganization, suggesting that nuclear hormone receptors are shapers of chromatin structure besides their known role of transcription factors.[51]

Glucocorticoid Receptors, Neurotransmitter, and Innate Immune Systems in Brain Disease

GCs enter the brain and bind to MRs and GRs. MRs have the function to maintain integrity and stability of limbic circuits and play a potential role in maintaining homeostasis,[52] while GRs play a reactive role in stress response, facilitate recovery of brain, distribute energy and maintain circulating levels of cortisol within normality through inhibition of HPA axis.[53] The brain has its own innate immune response, which is activated in response to both central and systemic immune challenges.[54] Inflammatory signals are known to act on the brain through key behavior-modulating multiple neurotransmitter systems, including serotonin, norepinephrine and dopamine. Activation of brain-neurotransmitters in turn activate pro-inflammatory cytokines, including IL-6 and TNFalfa, which influence the social and affective neural processes that induce depressed mood. GCs play a major role in the response of the brain to inflammatory stress, which depends on an NF-kB signal transduction pathway. Sleep loss induces increases in cellular and genomic markers of inflammation such as IL-6, TNFalpha.[55] Parenchymal microglia may produce elevated levels of molecules of the innate system such as IL-6, TNFalfa, and IL-1 beta, that can induce cell death in neuro-degenerative processes.[56] It has been hypothesized that the majority of psychiatric diseases are associated with the chronic degeneration of astroglia, which compromise brain homeostatic and defensive capability in diseases like schizophrenia and major depression disorders.[57] Research findings suggest a complex tightly balanced system in the brain and periphery that translates the effect of stress on specific tissues. Serious challenge to human capacity to adapt is associated with multiple morbidities, including heart disease, stroke, hypertension, diabetes, depression, obesity, and metabolic syndrome. Inflammation highly contributes to these comorbidities.[58]

Glucocorticoid Receptor Resistance

GC effect is ultimately determined at the level of the GR. Tissue sensitivity to GC differs among individuals, within tissues of the same individual, and within the same cells.[59] A reduced GR expression or binding affinity to its ligand, nuclear translocation, DNA binding or interaction with other transcription factors (NF-kB, AP-1), can lead to a state of GRs resistance.[60-61] Epigenetic changes in GR gene resulting in early life behavioral program have been shown in rats and humans.[62-63] GR is a severe problem associated with various inflammatory diseases.

Environmental factors that can induce GR resistance include chronic inflammation, exposure to infectious agents, chronic exposure to GCs. A decreased GR sensitivity to GCs has been shown in immune cells of HIV infected individuals.[64] Repeated social defeat induces GR resistance in macrophages. Epigenetic regulation such as DNA methylation and micro RNA expression may play a role in inducing glucocorticoid resistance.[65] GR resistance may also occur in asthma, rheumatoid arthritis, inflammatory bowel disease, and psoriasis, thyroiditis, lupus-like autoimmune syndrome.[66] GR resistance is also found in the induction phase of anti-leukemia therapy, in non-lymphoid malignancy, and in humans small cell lung carcinoma cell lines.[67] Insufficient GCs signaling resulting from decreased hormone bioavailability or reduced GR sensitivity may have devastating effects on body function. Such effects might be related in part to the role of glucocorticoids to restraining activation of the immune system and other components of the stress response. Stress-related neuropsychiatric disorders, associated with immune system activation/inflammation, may contribute to stress-related pathology, including alteration in behavior, insulin, cortisol sensitivity, and acquired immune responses.[68] Glucocorticoid resistance via impaired GR function reduces inhibitory feedback of HPA axis in inflammatory response, so influencing stress-related illness such as depression, metabolic syndrome, cardiovascular disease and osteoporosis, having inflammation as a common final pathway.

Obesity and the Metabolic Syndrome: The Role of Inflammation

The incidence of obesity is rising steadily throughout the world. Obesity has damaging effects on many organ systems; many of the co-morbid conditions are related to a metabolic syndrome characterized by large waist measure, high triglyceride levels, glucose intolerance, hypertension, and risk factors for the development of type-2 diabetes mellitus, systemic hypertension, coronary heart diseases, and heart failure. The incidence of respiratory disease, gastro-intestinal and musculo-skeletal disorders, thrombo-embolism, stroke, and cancer are increased with obesity.[69] Unhealthy eating habits, lack of exercise, and chronic stress as well as chronic inflammation have been considered causes of obesity and its pathological manifestation. Chronic stress has been associated with altered hormone secretion such as hypersecretion of cortisol and catecholamines, pro-inflammatory cytokines, as well as changes in circadian rhythm with evening elevation of cortisol[70] at a time during which the sensitivity of tissue to glucocorticoids is increased. This initiates a process that leads to accumulation of total but mostly visceral fat.

Environmental factors, unbalanced maternal nutrition, and an altered feeding behavior during the period of early development have also been suspected to lead to obesity. Stress and the early-life nutritional habit can affect the brain development leading to abnormal feeding behavior and neuro-endocrine alterations long-term.[71] Recent evidence has demonstrated alterations in epigenetic status following manipulation of nutrient environment during the developmental period.[72] Early life environment, if stressful, can have a life-long influence on these mechanisms, leading to hyperactive HPA axis and high cortisol plasma levels. HPA axis activation was found in adults of both sexes with low birth weight. Interestingly, alterations in DNA methylation of genes involved in cortisol regulation are present in adulthood in association with cardio-metabolic risk.[73]

All these data suggest that the neuro-endocrine-immune function might be damaged long before the METS onset. Studies have demonstrated that both obesity and metabolic disorders are associated with poorer cognitive performance, cognitive decline, and dementia. Further, there is a clear association between psychiatric medicine and significant weight gain.[74] There is growing understanding of a role of hypothalamic pituitary-adrenal axis dysfunction and basal systemic low-grade inflammation in the relationship between psychiatry and obesity. Both hypertrophied adipocytes and adipose tissue-resident lymphocytes and macrophages contribute to increasing circulating levels of pro-inflammatory cytokines, including TNFalfa, and important feeding relating peptides such as leptin and resistin, plasminogen activator inhibitor-1, C-reactive protein, interleukins IL-1 beta and IL-6 in obese individuals.[75]

Although evidence strongly suggests that GC action has a central role in METS, the state of GC excess is rare and the circulating level of cortisol is normal in the majority of patients with obesity and METS.[76] Then it was postulated that an elevated local regeneration of active glucocorticoids by 11ß-HSD1 may be an important factor in the development of complications associated with METS.[77] However, subsequent clinical trials with selective inhibitors compounds of

11beta HSD-1 showed only very moderate effect at high drug dose on diabetes and metabolic syndrome, and pre-clinical studies were interrupted.[78]

Metabolism, like inflammation, has complex control mechanisms. Nuclear receptors are among the most important regulators of metabolism and inflammation.[79] Moreover, nuclear receptors can both affect and be affected by reactive oxygen intermediate (ROI) and nitrogen intermediate (RNI) that have dual function in influencing both metabolism and inflammation in obesity. Glucocorticoid receptors and gonadal steroid receptors have similar capacity to produce epigenomic reorganization in adipose cells in addition to their well-established role as transcription factors.[79]

The increased number of macrophages that infiltrates obese adipose tissue, along with other cells of the stroma, also contribute to production of inflammatory cytokines.[80] During early diet induced obesity, there is an adaptive overproduction of vaso-dilators called adipocyte-derived relaxing factors (ADRF) that occurs in perivascular adipose tissue (PVAT). Under physiological conditions PVAT release a number of vasoactive substances such as ADRF, adiponectine, angiotensin, leptin, and nitric oxide that elicit a net beneficial anti-contractile effect on vascular function and are essential for the maintenance of vascular resistance.[81] However, in established obesity, PVAT loses its anti-contractile properties by an increase of contractile, oxidative, and inflammatory factors leading to endothelial dysfunction and vascular disease.[82] Weight loss by a different approach, including bariatric surgery by gastric bypass, significantly correlates with improvement in blood pressure levels, left ventricular mass, exercise capacity, and glucose tolerance. Thus, chronic inflammation appears to be a clinically important change that occurs in adipose tissue of subjects who become obese. Interestingly, expansion of fat without inflammation does not exert systemic metabolic effects such as systemic insulin resistance.[83] Insulin resistance has a key role in the pathogenesis of the metabolic syndrome; it leads to an increased oxidative stress, mitochondrial dysfunction, DNA damage, and cell death. Insulin suppresses endogenous production of glucose while controregulatory hormones such as cortisol and glucagon increase endogenous glucose production. Glucocorticoids increase gluconeo-genesis and blunt the suppressive effect of insulin on endogenous glu-cose production. The mechanisms by which glucocorticoids inhibit insulin activity are still not clear; however, studies on animals suggest an impairment of insulin-signaling cascade, leading to a reduced acti-vation of insulin target protein and genes in liver cells. Modifications that impair the action of insulin can be triggered by cytokines, such as TNFs, indicating that immune mediators can have a crucial regula-tory role in the glucose homeostasis.[84]

Emerging data demonstrate pivotal roles for brain insulin resis-tance and insulin deficiency as mediators of cognitive impairments and neuro-degeneration, particularly in Alzheimer disease.[85] Other inflammatory pathways are induced by cytoplasmatic organelle stress owing to nutrient overload resulting in metabolic stress. In these cases, activation of kinase such as JUN N. terminal kinase (JNK), and IK kinase-beta (IKKbeta) leads to metabolic alterations.[8] One such organelle, the endoplasmic reticulum (ER), has been shown to integrate inflammation and stress signal with metabolic status of cells, disruption of which results in disease such as type-2 diabetes.[86] Organelle stress in the inflammation contributes to the development of both obesity-associated insulin resistance and chronic metabolic disease. Metabolic and inflammatory pathways may converge at many levels of the organisms, including the levels of cells-surface receptors, nuclear intracellular chaperones, and nuclear receptors. These molec-ular sites allow for the coordination between nutrient and immune response in order to maintain homeostasis under diverse metabolic, immune conditions. Although low grade inflammation is a known pathological component of obesity, other triggering factors have actu-ally been identified. For example, gut-microbiota have been shown to have a role in the initiation of obesity and insulin resistance.[87]

Steroid hormones and their receptor signals that potentially modify body fat set-point include estrone, progesterone, aldosterone, retinoids, hydroxycalciferols, and especially their hormone receptors. The role of steroid hormones in obesity has been discussed by Alemany M.[88] A high prevalence of METS was shown in men with testosterone deficiency or treated with testosterone receptor antagonist.[89]

In conclusion, obesity may result from a combination of dysfunction of brain circuits and neuro-endocrine hormones related to pathological over-heating, physical inactivity, and other pathological conditions. It is increasingly appreciated that perinatal events can set an organism on a life-long trajectory for either health or disease, resilience or risk. Extensive research has documented the effects across the life span of over-nutrition, with strong links for an increased risk for obesity, metabolic, endocrine, and immune disorders as well as adverse mental health outcomes.

HIV Infection

It has been noted that during HIV infection, activated immune cells secrete pro-inflammatory cytokines that stimulate the release of systemic glucocorticoids. The triggering of this regulatory loop during inflammatory processes usually provides an important control over the immune system. This did not occur in HIV infected patients that showed an impressive increase of Th-directed cellular immune response in spite of an elevated level of cortisol, suggesting a cortisol resistance syndrome.[64,90] Treatment of these patients with HAART determines a dramatic decline of HIV and immune deficiency–related cause of death, but suppression of HIV replication by HAART is not associated with a reconstitution of the immune function, and this may account for unresolved inflammation in such patients.[91] This may lead to a cluster of conditions such as hypertension, high insulinemia, insulin resistance, dyslipidemia, fat redistribution, and increased risk of cardio-vascular diseases, stroke, diabetes, and neuro-cognitive and metabolic brain disorders. HIV-associated neuro-cognitive disorders (HAND) are potential consequences of HIV infection, and about half of adults with AIDS suffer from neurological complications related to HIV-1. HAND includes a spectrum of neurological disorders ranging from an asymptomatic form of neuro-cognitive impairments to an intermediate form and the severe form of HIV-associated dementia.

The increased life span of treated patients results in a chronic exposure of the brain to HIV-1 virions and viral proteins leading to inflammation as well as a concomitant chronic inflammation in the peripheral immune system leading to further neurological damage.[92] Chronic HIV-viral infection causes life-long antigenic stimulation and the development of a population of differentiated apoptosis-resistant, senescent T-cells, with limited proliferative potential.[93] This phenomenon is dysregulated in part by the regressive state of telomeres, the repeated DNA sequences that cap the ends of the chromosomes.[94] Reduction in telomere length influences the activity of P53 tumor suppressor pathways, apoptosis, and cell senescence.[95] Chronic inflammation may be the most important candidate for telomere length disturbances. In states of inflammation, increases in oxidative stress and cellular division may lead to the accelerated erosion of telomeres, crucial genomic structures that protect chromosomes from decay.[96] The final result is an immune system of a limited capacity to recognize novel antigens and hence to prevent disease. HAART treatment is also associated with activation of MR and renin angiotensin aldosterone system, which have hypertensive and pro-inflammatory effects; however, the usefulness of MR antagonists is limited. Efforts are underway to selectively modulate glucocorticoids, mineralocorticoids receptors, and other nuclear receptors. This is facilitated by structural function similarities of these receptors.[97]

Discussion

As modern society is troubled by complex multifactorial disease, research is called to govern complex realities, including unresolved inflammation, cancer, obesity, and metabolic syndrome and its detrimental cardiovascular complications, as well as depression and other heterogeneous brain disorders.

The brain is the central organ of stress and of adaptation to stressors because it perceives what are threatening or potentially threatening factors and initiates behavioral and physiological response to those challenges. However, it also is a target of stressful experiences and of the hormones and other mediators of the stress response.

In the response to a stressful encounter, the brain activates a complex stress system that engages the organism in an adaptive response to the threatening situation. The adaptive response acts on multiple peripheral tissues and on feedback to the brain. Diseases can occur when the balance between multiple players such as behavioral, neuro-endocrine-immune-metabolic systems, and responsive tissues is upset, so that the adaptive systems convert into a maladapted, detrimental chain of events. It is under these conditions that inflammatory control mechanisms are engaged. The problem with inflammation is not how often it starts, but how often it fails to subside. Unresolved inflammation is not the primary cause of major and more frequent chronic diseases, such as cancer, brain disease, obesity, and HIV infection, but it contributes significantly to their pathogenesis.

Epigenetic mechanisms are dominant mechanisms for the transduction of environmental inputs such as stress and inflammation into lasting physiological and behavioral changes, and the development of neuro-psychiatric diseases.

Stress has a number of known effects on epigenetic marks in the brain, producing alterations in DNA methylation and histone modifications in most of the stress-sensitive brain regions, including the hippocampus, amygdala, and pre-frontal cortex.[98–99] It has been shown that both acute and chronic stress are altered by methylation of histone. One of the key players in stress is the corticoid hormone receptor family, which affects brain functioning through both delayed genomic and rapid non-genomic mechanisms. Nuclear receptors (NR) superfamily governs diverse biological processes as development, physiology, and disease. Glucocorticoid nuclear receptors play an essential role in the response to environmental stressors. A number of diseases including autoimmune, infectious, and inflammatory disorders as well as certain neuro-psychiatric disorders, such as major depression, have been associated to a decreased responsiveness to glucocorticoids, which is believed to be related to impaired functioning of the glucocorticoid receptors. Glucocorticoid resistance may be a result of impaired GR function, secondary to exposure to inflammatory cytokines as may occur during chronic medical illness.[100]

Nuclear hormone receptors in general are significant shapers of chromatin structure, in addition to their role as transcription factors. Chronic inflammation associated with immune-mediated disease represents a profound stress factor for the immune system affecting cellular-turnover, replication, and exhaustion. Immune cell longevity is tightly connected to the functional integrity of telomeres, which are regulated by cell multiplication, exposure to oxidative stress, and DNA repair mechanism. The loss of the immune function in aging is associated with conditions that limit life span, such as infectious susceptibility and malignancy.[101] Telomeres are the natural end of linear chromosomes, and function to cap chromosomal ends. Short telomeres force the cells to enter into senescence or apoptotic death. Tissues under permanent replicative stress, and brain cells' ability to build memory, are particularly dependent on cell survival. Notably, chronic infection accelerates erosion of the cell telomeres in immune cells through increased proliferative stress. Reduction of telomeric length of PBMCs seems to be a predictor for progression of atherosclerotic disease, myocardial infarction, and reduction in left ventricular mass. Telomere length has been connected to cancer incidence and cancer mortality.[102] Reduction in telomere length influences the activity of P53 tumor suppressor pathways, malignant cell transformation, apoptosis, and cell senescence.[95] For reasons that remain merely defined, long-term treated HIV persons have a shortened life span, which is linked to an increased risk of complications, including heart, cancer, liver, kidney, and bone disease and neuro-cognitive decline. This phenomenon is regulated in part by the progressive reduction in telomere length. Notably, patients with type-1 diabetes mellitus (DM) present a reduction in telomeric length in arterial cells. Such reduction correlated strongly with the HbA1C concentration. In addition, telomeric length in arteries and mononuclear cells of patients with uncontrolled DM were significantly shorter than telomeres in mononuclear cells of patients with well-controlled DM.[103]

The development of strategies that slow down the loss of immune function with progressive cell age has the potential to afford novel therapeutic avenues for a number of degenerative diseases and modifies epigenetic marks contributing to disease developing. Epigenetic silencing of gene transcription by methylation of DNA or modifications of histones is a key event in neoplastic initiation and progression. Alterations in the epigenome have been identified in virtually all types of cancer and involve multiple genes and molecular pathways. It has been proposed that epigenic gene-disregulation may represent a first step in tumor genesis, possibly by affecting the normal differentiation of stem cells and predisposing the cells to additional oncogenic insults. Aberrant DNA methylation and histone acetylation has been linked to a number of age-related disorders, including cancers, obesity, metabolic syndrome, type-2 diabetes, autoimmune disorders, and others. Since epigenetic alterations are reversible, modifying epigenetic marks contributing to disease development may provide an approach to designing new therapies.[104] Inhibitors of DNA-methyl transferases or histone diacetilases have been approved for clinical use.[105]

Therapeutic Interventions

Mesenchymal stem cells (MSCs) represent a promising tool for treatment of chronic inflammatory diseases. MSCs appear to suppress inflammation through secretion of anti-inflammatory cytokines such as IL-10 and GFbeta,[106] interferon-gamma,[107] soluble human leucocytes antigen-G 92, L-1 receptors agonist,[108] and expression of immune regulatory enzymes such as cyclo-oxigenase and indolamine 2,3 deoxy-genase.[109] MSCs inhibit immune globuline production and arrest B-lymphocytes cell cycle. They also interfere with dendritic cell differentiation, maturation, and function. Based on these properties, MSCs have been used in regenerative medicine, for the treatment of autoimmune diseases,[110,111] and for inhibiting tumor proliferation. MSCs are now used as an easy-to-harvest tool for cell therapy and exhibit robust multipotency and multilineage potential in vitro. Despite these attractive features, MSCs also undergo significant senescence and decline in multipotency expression after multiple passages in culture.[112,113] These findings raise cautionary notes whenever long-passaged MSCs are used in a clinical setting and prompt the need for novel approaches that may oppose senescence and optimize the expression of multipotency in such a promising tool for cell therapy.

Recent studies demonstrated that the exposed MSCs in the presence of Zebrafish growth and differentiation factors harvested at different developmental stages showed that only the late (20 somites and pharingula) developmental stage factors had significantly decreased cell proliferation and viability. These factors determined the activation of a differentiation or proapoptotic program, as shown by the derangement in nuclear morphology and the chromatin condensation, and by the activation of the cascade of caspases. For these reasons the factors taken from these late stages of differentiation of the Zebrafish embryo are used to control tumor growth[114,115,116,117,118,119,120,121] in the clinical treatment of patients, first of all patients affected by hepatocellular carcinoma.[122,123] These factors are also used to slow down the high speed of multiplication of cheratinocites in psoriasis.[124] Otherwise, the factors of the first stages of development (middle-blastula-gastrula, tail bud, 5 somites) did not induce MSCs apoptosis, nor did they decrease cell viability. This contrasting behavior may result from a fine equilibrium between first stages-induced transcription of Oct-4, Sox-2, TERT, Bmi-1, and c-Myc, known to inhibit apoptotic pathways and the increase in Bax/Bcl-2 mRNA ratio observed in the first stages-exposed MSCs.[125]

During Zebrafish embryogenesis, the expression of the pluripo-tency genes Pou5f1/Oct-4 and Sox-2 is timely regulated by defined factors that are mainly restricted to the early developmental pattern (during the first hpf).[126,127,128] Our data show that MSCs are able to selectively respond to factors restricted to the very early, but not late, developmental stages of Zebrafish embryo with a transcriptional increase in the same two stemness-related genes necessary for the expression of family members of transcription factors that contribute to the maintenance of human stem cell pluripotency and self-renewal. The overexpression of stemness genes elicited by the first stages of cell differentiation factors was paralleled by an increase in the tran-scription of both Bmi-1 and TERT. Notably, these findings indicate that both genes exert a major role in counteracting aging processes in vivo and cell senescence in vitro. Bmi-1 is emerging as a major aging repressor and is transcriptionally down-regulated when cells undergo replicative senescence.[129] TERT opposes cell senescence by counteract-ing telomere shortening.[130] Studies on brain development in mice have correlated a decrease in TERT expression and activity with decreased neuroblast proliferation and differentiation. Moreover, it has been demonstrated that MSCs or bone marrow stromal stem cells lack-ing telomerase activity undergo premature cellular senescence, with a progressive decline in the expression of early mesenchymal stem cell markers.

The maintenance of stemness gene expression is also important in the prevention of cell senescence. The singular loss of the Bright/Arid3A transcription factor, the founding member of the ARID fam-ily of transcriptions factors, which binds directly to the promoter/enhancer regions of Oct-4, Sox-2, contributing to their repression in both mouse embryonic fibroblasts (MEFs) and mouse embryonic stem cells (ESCs), was found to bypass the cell senescence barrier, leading to MEF reprogramming.[131, 132] We show for the first time that human stem cell exposure to early developmental stage of Zebrafish embryo stem cell growth and differentiation factors may represent a useful tool to enhance stem cell expression of multipotency and activate both telomerase-dependent and -independent antagonists of cell senescence. In addition we describe in another article of this special issue that the mix of all stages of cell differentiation taken from Zebrafish embryos are able to prevent in a very significant way the neuro-degeneration of the cell of the hippocampus.

All these effects were obtained without gene manipulation through viral vector mediated gene transfer, or expensive synthetic chemistry. In conclusion, we can say that exposure to early developmental stage of Zebrafish embryo growth and differentiation factors may enhance stem cell expression of multipotency and activate both telomerase-dependent and -independent antagonists of cell senescence. These outcomes may prove rewarding during prolonged expansion in culture, as it occurs in most cell therapy protocols. These factors can also be used as anti-aging factors in old patients in clinical use. In the opposite direction, the factors taken from the late stages of cell differentiation of Zebrafish embryo can be used to control cell proliferation of tumor cells and to slow down the high speed of multiplication of cheratinocites as it happens in psoriasis and in many other diseases. Finally, all the network of factors present in all stages of cell differentiation can be used to prevent neuro-degeneration and other degenerative phenomena in chronic diseases and to maintain the homeostasis of the organism under stress and under consequences of stress phenomena (strain).

Conclusion

Complex signal transduction pathways govern regulated development processes of multi-cellular embryos. Aberrant regulation and transduction of embryonal pathways has been implicated in birth defect, alterations in tissue regeneration, stem cell renewal, and cancer growth.[133] This might explain vulnerability of most traits of human anatomy and physiology that negatively affect homeostasis. Disruption of homeostatic mechanisms due to the impact of acute life-style and genetic background and early life environment can have a life-long influence on neuro-endocrine mechanisms connecting stress to immune response and metabolism and leads to chronic activation of inflammatory mechanisms. Serious challenge to human capacity to adapt is associated with multiple morbidity, including heart disorders, stroke, hypertension, diabetes, metabolic syndrome, cancer, HIV infection, and neuro-degenerative disease.

Epigenetic mechanisms are considered essential for the transduction of environmental stress experiences into chronic inflammatory diseases, leaving traces expressed in the genome. Acute and chronic stress are altered by DNA methylation and histone modifications in stress-sensitive brain regions that may contribute to neuro-degenerative disorders. Aberrant DNA methylation and histone acetylation have been also linked to a number of disorders, including cancer, obesity, metabolic syndrome, type-2 diabetes, and autoimmune disorders. Nuclear receptors are among the most important regulators of metabolism and inflammation: they play an essential role in the response to environmental stressors. Reduced sensitivity of glucocorticoid receptors, induced by epigenetic changes, may lead to cortisol resistance status that has devasting effects on body function involving excessive deterioration of immune and metabolic functions. Glucocorticoid receptors and gonadal steroid receptors have similar capacity to produce epigenomic reorganization in dipose cells in addition to their established role as transcription factors.

Efforts are underway to modulate selectively glucocorticoids, mineralocorticoid receptors, and other nuclear receptors. This is facilitated by the structural function similarities of these receptors.

Chronic infection has been shown to accelerate erosion of telomeres in immune cells. Such alterations have been connected with cancer induction and mortality and changes in P53 tumor suppressor pathways influencing malignant transduction, apoptosis, and cell senescence. Reduction of telomere length has been also observed in long-term treated HIV patients and in type-1 diabetes mellitus, and it is associated with increased risks of severe metabolic, vascular, and brain disturbances.

The final result of non-genomic alterations just described is an immune system of limited capacity to recognize novel antigens and hence to prevent chronic degenerative disorders. Since epigenetic alterations are reversible, modifying epigenetic marks contributing to disease development may provide an approach to design new therapies. We propose here an epigenetic treatment of chronic inflammatory and degenerative diseases using stem cell differentiation stage factors of Zebrafish embryos taken at the final stages of cell differentiation to induce cell differentiation, slow down proliferation of cancer cells, or of cheratinocites in psoriasis. On the contrary we can use stem cell differentiation factors taken at the early stages of cell differentiation to enhance stemness genes and multi-potency, activate both telomerase dependent and independent antagonist of cells senescence, and favor in this way the regeneration of tissues.

Our aim now is to provide novel insights regarding the potential combination of epigenetic reprogramming mechanisms in controlling plasticity and pluripotencies of stem cell populations, and define stem cells differentiation factors capable of repairing different pathological stem cells at the origin of numerous chronic diseases.

References

1. Steiman, L. Elaborate interactions between the immune and nervous systems. *Nat. Immunol.* 2004, 5:575–581.
2. Dantzer, R.; Bluthé, R. M.; Layé, S.; Bret-Dibat, J. L.; Parnet, P.; Kelley, K. W. Cytokines and sickness behavior. Ann N Y *Acad Sci.* 1998, 1;840: 586–90.
3. Dantzer, R.; Konsman, J. P.; Bluthé, R. M.; Kelley, K. W. Neural and humoral pathways of communication from the immune system to the brain: parallel or convergent? *Auton. Neurosci.* 2000, 85(1–3): 60–5.
4. Watkins, L. R.; Maier, SF.; Goehler, L. E. Cytokine-to-brain communication: A review & analysis of alternative mechanisms. *Life Sci.* 1995, 57(11): 1011–26.
5. Hopkins, S. J.; Rothwell, N. J. Cytokines and the nervous system. Expression and recognition. *Trends neurosci.* 1995, 18: 83–88.

6. Soltow, Q. A.; Johns, D. P.; Promislow, D. E. A network perspective on metabolism and aging. *Integr. Comp.Biol.* 2010, 50: 844–54.

7. Taniguchi, C. M.; Emanuelli, B.; Kahn, C. R. Critical nodes in signaling pathways: insights into insulin action. *Nat Rev Mol Cell Biol.* 2006, 7(2): 85–96.

8. Hotamisligil, G. S. Inflammation and metabolic disorders. *Nature.* 2006, 44: 860–867.

9. Hotamisligil, G. S.; Erbay, E. Nutrient sensing and inflammation in metabolic diseases. *Nat Rev Immunol.* 2008, 8; 923–934.

10. Libby, P. Inflammation and cardiovascular disease mechanisms. *Am. J. Clin Nut.* 2006, 83: 456S–460S.

11. Trinchieri, G. Cancer and inflammation: an old intuition with rapidly evolving new concepts. *Annu. Rev. Immunol.* 2012, 30: 677–706.

12. Wyss-Coray, T.; Mucke, L. Inflammation in neurodegenerative disease—a double-edged sword. *Neuron.* 2002, 35: 419–32.

13. de Kloet, E. R.; Joëls, M.; Holsboer, F. Stress and the brain: from adaptation to disease. *Nat Rev Neurosci.* 2005, 6(6): 463–75.

14. Straub, R. H.; Del Rey, A.; Basedowsky, H. O. Emerging concepts for the pathogenesis of chronic disabling inflammatory diseases: neuro-endocrine-immune interactions and evolutionary biology. In Ader, R., ed. *Psychoneuro immunology.* San Diego, CA: Elsevier-Academic Press, 2007, 217–32.

15. Okin, D.; Medzhitov, R. Evolution of inflammatory diseases. *Current Biol.* 2012, 225 R733–40.

16. Baffy, G.; Loscalzo. J. Complexity and network dynamics in physiological adaptation: an integrated view. *Physiology and behavior* 2014, 131: 49–56.

17. Schreiber, RD.; Old, LJ.; Smyth, MJ. Cancer Immunoediting: Integrating immunities' roles in cancer suppression and promotion. *Sci.* 2011, 331 (6024): 1565–1570.

18. Vasely, MD.; Kershow, MH.; Schreiber, RD. Natural innate and adaptive immunity to cancer. *Annu. Rev. Immunol.* 2011, 29(1): 235–271.

19. Shin, MS.; Kim, HS.; Lee, SH. Mutations of tumor necrosis factor-related apoptosis-including ligand receptor-1 and receptor-2 genes in metastatic breast cancer. *Cancer res.* 2001, 61: 4942–4946.

20. Jiang, X.; Shapiro, DJ. The immune system and the inflammation in breast cancer, *Mol.cell.endocrinol* 2014, 382(1): 673–682.

21. Mantovani, A.; Romero, P.; Palucka, AK.; Marincola, FM. Tumor immunity:

effector response to tumor and role of the microenvironment. *Lance* 2008, 371(9614): 771–83. doi: 10.1016 /S0140–6736(08)60241–X.

22. Schetter, A. J.; Heegaard, N. H.; Harris, C. C. Inflammation and cancer: inter-weaving microRNA, free radical, cytokine and p53 pathways. *Carcinogenesis* 2010, 31(1):37–49. doi: 10.1093/carcin/bgp272.

23. Pan, J. S.; Hong,M. Z.; Ren, J. L. Reactive oxygen species: a double-edged sword in oncogenesis. *World J Gastroenterol.* 2009, 14;15(14): 1702–7.

24. Hussain, S. P.; Harris CC. Inflammation and cancer: an ancient link with novel potentials. *Int. J Cancer* 2007, 1;121(11): 2373–80.

25. Kisley, L. R.; Barrett, B. S.; Bauer, A. K.; Dwyer-Nield, L. D.; Barthel, B.; Meyer, A. M.; Thompson, D. C.; Malkinson, A. M. Genetic ablation of induc-ible nitric oxide synthase decreases mouse lung tumorigenesis. *Cancer Res.* 2002, 1;62(23): 6850–6.

26. Grivennikov, S.; Karin, E.; Terzic, J.; Mucida, D.; Yu, G. Y.; Vallabhapurapu, S.; Scheller, J.; Rose-John, S.; Cheroutre, H.; Eckmann, L.; Karin, M. IL-6 and Stat3 are required for survival of intestinal epithelial cells and development of colitis-associated cancer. *Cancer Cell* 2009, 3;15(2):103–13. doi: 10.1016 /j.ccr.2009.01.001.

27. Mosser, D. M.; Zhang X. Interleukin-10: new perspectives on an old cytokine. *Immunol Rev.* 2008, 226:205–18. doi: 10.1111/j.1600-065X.2008.00706.x.

28. Lu, L. F; Liston, A. MicroRNA in the immune system, microRNA as an immune system. *Immunology* 2009, 127(3):291–8. doi: 10.1111/j.1365-2567 .2009.03092.x.

29. Rius, J.; Guma, M.; Schachtrup, C.; Akassoglou, K.; Zinkernagel, A. S.; Nizet, V.; Johnson, R. S.; Haddad, G. G.; Karin, M. NF-kappaB links innate immunity to the hypoxic response through transcriptional regulation of HIF-1alpha. *Nature* 2008, 453(7196):807–11. doi: 10.1038/nature06905. Epub 2008 Apr 23.

30. Balkwill, F. Tumor necrosis factor and cancer. *Nat Rev Cancer* 2009, 9(5): 361–71. doi: 10.1038/nrc2628. Epub 2009 Apr 3.

31. Popivanova, BK.; Kitamura, K.; Wu, Y.; Kondo,T.; Kagaya,T.; Kaneko, S.; Oshima, M.; Fujii, C.; Mukaida N. Blocking TNF-alpha in mice reduces colorectal carcinogenesis associated with chronic colitis. *J Clin Invest.* 2008, 118(2): 560–70. doi: 10.1172/JCI32453.

32. Kulbe, H.; Thompson, R.; Wilson, JL.; Robinson, S.; Hagemann, T.; Fatah, R.; Gould, D.; Ayhan, A.; Balkwill F. The inflammatory cytokine tumor necrosis factor-alpha generates an autocrine tumor-promoting network

in epithelial ovarian cancer cells. *Cancer Res.* 2007, 15;67(2): 585–92.

33. Basu S.; Nachat-Kappes R.; Caldefie-Chézet, F.; Vasson M. P. Eicosanoids and adipokines in breast cancer: from molecular mechanisms to clinical considerations, antioxidants & redox signaling. *Antioxid Redox Signal* 2013, 18(3): 323–360. doi:10.1089/ars.2011.4408.

34. Schreiber, R. D.; Old, L. J.; Smyth M. J. Cancer immunoediting: integrating immunity's roles in cancer suppression and promotion. *Science* 2011, 331(6024): 1565–70. doi: 10.1126/science.1203486.

35. Vesely, M. D.; Kershow, M. H.; Schreiber, R. D.; Smyth M. J. Natural innate and adaptive immunity to cancer. *Annu Rev. Immunol.* 2011, 29(1): 235–271. doi: 10.1146/annu rev-immunol-031210–101324.

36. Jiang, X.; Shapiro, D. J. The immune system and inflammation in breast cancer. *Mol Cell Endocrinol.* 2014, 382(1): 673–682. doi: 10.1016/j.mce.2013.06.003.

37. Jiang, X.; Ellison, S. J.; Alarid, Shapiro, D. J. Interplay between the levels of estrogen and estrogen receptors controls of the granzyme inhibitor, proteinase inhibitor-9 and susceptibility to immune surveillance by natural killer cells. *Oncogene* 2007, 26:4106–4114. doi:10.1038/sj.onc. 1210197.

38. Jiang, X. Harnessing the immune system for the treatment of breast cancer. J. of the Zhejiang University Sci. B (Biomed and Biotecnol) 2014,15(1): 1–15.

39. Rose, D. P.; Vona-Davis, L. The cellular and molecular mechanisms by which insulin influences breast cancer risks and progression. *Endocr. relat. cancer* 2012, 19(6): R225–41.

40. Crujeiras, A. B.; Diaz-Lagares, A.; Carreira, M. C. Oxidative stress associated to dysfunctional adipose tissue : a potential link between obesity, type-2 diabetes mellitus and breast cancer. *Free radic research* 2013, 47(4): 243–56.

41. Woo, H. D.; Kim, J. Global DNA hypomethylation in peripheral blood leucocytes as a bio-marker for cancer risk. a meta-analysis. PLoS 1 2012, 7(4): e34–615.

42. Yu, I. C.; Lin, H. I.; Sparks, J. D.; Yen, S.; Chang, C. Androgen receptors role in insulin resistance and obesity in males: the linkage of androgen-deprivation therapy to metabolic-syndrome. *Diabetes* 2014, 63(10): 3180–8.

43. Nyquist, M. D.; Dehm, SM. Interplay between genomic alterations and androgen receptors signaling during prostate cancer development and progression. *Horm Canc.* 2013, 4: 61–69. doi:10. 1007/s 12672-013-0131-4.

44. Carruba, G. Estrogen and prostate cancer: an eclipsed truth in an androgen-dominated scenario. *J Cell Biochem.* 2007, 102(4): 899–911.

45. Zhu, P.; Baek, S. H.; Bourk, E. M.; Ohgi, K. A.; Garcia-Bassets, I.; Sanjo, H.; Akira, S.; Kotol, P. F.; Glass, C. K.; Rosenfeld,M. G.; Rose D. W. Macrophage/cancer cell interactions mediate hormone resistance by a nuclear receptor derepression pathway. *Cell* 2006,124, 615–629.

46. Gross, K. L.; Cydlowsky, J. A. Tissue-specific glucocorticoid action: a family affair. *Trends Endocrinol.Metab.* 2008, 19: 331–339.

47. Oakley, R. H.; Cydlowsky, J. A. Homologous down regulation of the glucocorticoid receptor: the molecular machinery. *Crit Rev Eukaryot Gene Expr.* 1993, 3(2): 63–88.

48. Levin, E. R. Rapid signaling by steroid receptors. Regulatory, integrative and comparative physiology. *American Journal of Physiology* 2008, 295 R 1425-R1430 doi: 10.1152/ajpregu.90605.2008.

49. Hammes, S. R. & Levin, E. R. Extranuclear steroid receptors: nature and actions. *Endocrine reviews* 2007; 28: 726–41.

50. Grossmann, C & Gekle, M. New aspect of rapid aldosterone signaling. *Molecular and cellular endocrinology* 2009, 308: 53–62.

51. Hunter, R. G.; Gagnidze, K.; McEwen, B.; Pfaff, D. W. Stress and the dynamic genoma: steroids, epigenetics and the transposome. *Proc Natl Acad Sci U.S.A.* 2014, pii: 201411260.

52. Joëls, M. Functional actions of corticosteroids in the hippocampus. *European Journal of Pharmacology* 2008, 583: 312–321.

53. De Kloet, E. R.; Reul, G. M. Feedback action and tonic influence of corticosteroids on brain function: a concept arising from the heterogeneity of brain receptor systems. *Psycho neuroendocrinology* 1987, 12: 83–105.

54. Glezer, I.; Rivest, S. Glucocorticoids: protectors of the brain during innate immune responses. *Neuroscientist* 2004, 10(6): 538–52.

55. Vgontzas, A. N.; Zoumakis, E.; Bixler, E. O.; Lin, H. M.; Follett, H.; Kales, A.; Chrousos, G. P. Adverse effects of modest sleep restriction on sleepiness, performance, and inflammatory cytokines. *J. Clin.Endocr.Metab.* 2004, 89: 2119–2126.

56. Scarano, F.; Baltuch, G. Microglia as mediators of inflammatory and degenerative diseases. *Annu. Rev. Neurosci.* 1999, 22: 219–40.

57. Verkhzhsky, A.; Rodigue, S.; Stardo, L. Astroglia pathology: a central element of neuro psychiatric disease. *The Neuro Scientist* 2014, 20 (6) 576–578.

58. Nguyen, M. D.; Julien, J. P.; Rivest, S. Innate immunity: the missing link in neuro protection and neuro degeneration. *Nat. Rev. neurosci.* 2002, (3): 216–27.

59. Lauretsky, H.; Irwin, M. Resiliance and aging. *Aging health* 2007, 3: 309–323.

60. Chrousos, G. P. Stress and disorders. *Nat. Rev. Endocr.* 2009, 5: 374–381.

61. van Rossum, E. F.; van den Akker, E. L. Glucocorticoids resistance. *Endocr. Dev.* 2010, 20: 127–136.

62. Debosscher, K.; van den Berghe W.; Aegheman, G. Crosstalk between nuclear receptors and nuclear factor kB. *Oncogene* 2006, 25: 6868–6886.

63. Miller, A. H.; Maletic, V.; Raison, C. L. Inflammation and its discontent : the role of cytokines in the pathophysiology of major depression. *Biol. Psychiatry* 2009, 65(9): 732–741.

64. Norbiato, G.; Bevilacqua, M.; Vago, T.; Baldi, G.; Chebat, E.; Bertora, P.; Moroni, M.; Galli, M.; Oldenburg, N. Cortisol resistance in acquired immune deficiency syndrome, *J.Clin.Endocr.Metab.* 1992, 74(3): 608–13.

65. Yung, S. H.; Vang Y.; Kim, T.; Tarrav, R.; Reader, B.; Powel, N.; Sheridan, JF. Molecular mechanism of repeated social defeat induced glucocorticoid resistance. Role of the micro RNA. *Brain behavior and immunity* 2015, 195–206.

66. Yang, N.; Ray, D. W.; Matthews, L. C. Current concepts in glucocorticoid resistance. *Steroids* 2012, 77(11): 1041–9.

67. Balkwill, F. Tumor necrosis factor and cancer. *Nat. Rev. Cancer* 2009, 9: 361–371.

68. Raison, C. L.; Miller, A. H. When not enough is too much. *Am J. Psychiatry* 2003, 160 (9): 1554–65.

69. Haslam, D. W.; James, W. P. Obesity. *Lancet* 2005, 366(9492): 1197–209.

70. Nicolaides, N. C.; Kyratzi, E.; Lamprokostopoulou, A.; Chrousos, G. P.; Charmandari E. Stress, the stress system and the role of glucocorticoids. *Neuroimmunomodulation* 2015, 22(1–2): 6–19.

71. Spencer, S. J. Perinatal programming of neuroendocrine mechanisms connecting feeding behavior. *Stress frontiers in neurosciences* 2013, vol. 7 doi: 10.3389/Fnins.2013.00109.

72. Bruce, K. D.; Hanson, M. A. The developmental origins, mechanisms and implications of metabolic syndrome. *The journal of nutrition.* 2010, doi: 10.3945/JN.109.111179.

73. Reynolds R. M. Glucocorticoids excess and the developmental origin of disease: two decades of testing the hypothesis—2012 Curd Ricter Harward winner. *Psycho neuroendocrinology* 2013, 38(1): 1–11.

74. Nguyen, J. C. D.; Killcross, AS.; Jenkins, T. A. Obesity and cognitive decline: role of inflammation and vascular changes. *Front Neurosci.* 2014, doi: 10.3389/Fnins.2014.00375.

75. Ouchi, N.; Walsh, K.; Lugus, J. J.; Walsh, K. Adipokines in inflammation and metabolic disease. *Nat. Rev. Immunol.* 2011, 11(2): 85–97.

76. Anagnostis, P.; Athyros, V. G.; Tziomalos, K.; Karagiannis, A.; Mikhailidis, DP. The pathogenic role of cortisol in the metabolic syndrome: hypothesis. *J. Clin. Endocrinol. Metab.* 2009, 94: 2692–2701.

77. Stewart, P. M. Tissue specific cushing's syndrome 11Beta-hydroxy steroid dehydrogenases and the redefinition of corticosteroid hormone action. *Eur. J. Endocrinol.* 2003, 149: 163–168.

78. Scott, J. S.; Golberg, F. W.; Turnbull, AV. Medical chemistry of inhibitors of 11Beta-hydroxy-steroid dehydrogenase type-1. *J. Med. Chem.* 2014, 57: 4466–4486.

79. Nathan, C. Epidemic inflammation: pondering obesity. *Mol. Med.* 2008, 14(7–8): 485–92.

80. Tilg, H.; Moschen, A. R. Inflammatory mechanisms in the regulation of insulin resistance. *Mol. Med.* 2008, 14(3–4): 222–231.

81. Gollasch, M.; Dubrovska, G. Parachrine role for periadventitial adipose tissue in the regulation of arterial tone. *Trends Pharmacol. Sci.* 2004, Vol. 25, no. 12 pp 647–653.

82. Fernandez-Alfonso, MS.; Gill-Ortega, M.; Garcia-Prieto., C. F; Aranguez, I.; Ruiz-Gaio, M.; Somoza, B. Mechanisms of perivascular adipose tissue dysfunction in obesity. *International Journal of Endocrinol.* 2013, Vol. 2013. Art. I. D. 402053. Page 8. doi: 10.1155/2013/402053.

83. Kim, J. Y.; van de Wal, E.; Laplante, M.; Azara, A. Trujillo, M. E.; Hofmann, S. M. Obesity-associated improvement in metabolic profile through expansion of adipose tissue. *J. Clin. Invest.* 2007, 117(9): 2621–2637.

84. Peraldi, P.; Hotamisligil, G. S.; Buurman, W. A.; White, M. F.; Spiegelman, B. M. Tumor necrosis factor (TNF)-alpha inhibits insulin signaling through stimulation of the p55 TNF receptor and activation of sphingomyelinase. *J Biol Chem.* 1996, 271(22): 13018–22.

85. De la Monte, S. M. Insulin resistance and Alzheimer's disease. BMB reports 2009, 42(8): 475–481.

86. Ozcan, U.; Cao, Q.; Yilmaz, E.; Lee, A. H.; Iwakoshi, N. N.; Ozdelen, E.; Tuncman, G.; Görgün, C.; Glimcher, L. H.; Hotamisligil, G. S. Endoplasmic reticulum stress links obesity, insulin action, and type-2 diabetes. *Science* 2004, 306: 457–461.

87. Turnbaugh, P. J.; Ley, R. E.; Mahowald, M. A.; Magrini, V.; Mardis, E. R.; Gordon, J. I. An obesity-associated gut microbiome with increased capacity for energy harvest. *Nature* 2006, 444: 1027–1031.

88. Alemany, M. Do the interactions between the glucocorticoids and sex hormones regulate the development of the metabolic syndrome? *Front. Endocrinol.* 2012, 3: 27.

89. Garcia-Cruz, E.; Leiber Tamajo, A.; Romedo, J.; Piqueras, M.; Luque, P.; Cardenas, A. O.; Alcaraz, A. *J. Sex med* 2013, 10(10): 2529–38.

90. Norbiato, G.; Bevilacqua, M.; Vago, T.; Taddei, A.; Clerici, M. Glucocorticoids and the immune function in the human immunodeficiency virus infection: a study in hypercortisolemic and cortisol-resistant patients. *J Clin Endocrinol Metab.* 1997, 82(10):3260–3.

91. Norbiato, G. Endocrine, metabolic, and immunologic components of HIV infection. Ann N Y *Acad Sci.* 2012, 1262:51–5. doi: 10.1111/j.1749-6632.2012.06620.x.

92. Rao, V. R.; Ruiz, A. P.; Prasad, V. R. Viral and cellular factors underlying neuropathogenesis in HIV associated neurocognitive disorders. *AIDS Research and Therapy* 2014, 11: 13.

93. Effros, R. B.; Pawelek, G. Replicative senescence of T-cells : does the Hayflick limit lead to immune exhaustion? *Immunol. today* 1997, 18: 450–454.

94. Blackburn, E. H. Structure and function of telomeres. *Nature* 1991, 350: 569–573.

95. Campisi, J.; d'Adda, D.; Fagagna, F. Cellular senescence : when bad things happen to good cells. *Nat. Rev. Mol. Cell. Biol.* 2007, 8: 729–40.

96. Wong, J. Y.; De Vivo, I.; Lin, X.; Fang, S. C.; Christiani, D. C. The relationship between inflammatory biomarkers and telomere length in an occupational prospective cohort study. *PLoS One* 2014;9(1): e87348. doi: 10.1371/journal.pone.0087348. eCollection 2014.

97. Baxter, J. D.; Funder, J. W.; Apriletti, JW.; Webb, P. Toward selective modulating mineralocorticoid receptor function: lessons from other systems. *Mol cell endocrinol* 2004, 217 (1–2): 151–65.

98. Hunter, R. G.; McEwen, B. S. Stress and anxiety across the life span : structural plasticity and epigenetic regulation. *Epigenomics* 2013, 5(2): 177–194.

99. Hunter, R. G. Epigenetic effects of stress and corticosteroid in the brain. *Front. Cell. Neurosci.* 2012, 6: 18.

100. Leader, J. E.; Wang, C.; Fu, M.; Pestell, R. G. Epigenic regulation of nuclear steroid receptors. *Biochem. Pharmacol* 2006, 72(11): 1589–96.

101. Aubert, G.; Lansdorp, P. M. Telomeres and aging. *Physiol.Rev.* 2008, 88: 557–79.

102. Willeit, P.; Willeit J.; Majer, A.; Weger, S.; Oberhollenzer, F.; Brandstatter,

A.; Kronenberg, F; Kieckl, S. Telomere length and risk incidence cancer and cancer mortality. *JAMA* 2010, 304: 69–75.

103. Uziel, O.; Singer, JA.; Danicek, V.; Sahaar, G.; Berkov, E.; Lucihansky, M.; Fraser, A.; Ram, R.; Lahav, M. Telomeres dynamics in arteries and mono-nuclear cells in diabetes patients: effect of diabetes and of glycemic control. *Exp. Gerontol* 2007; 42: 971–8.

104. Lu, Q.; Qiu, X.; Hu, N.; Wen, H.; Su, Y.; Richardson, BC. Epigenetics, disease, and therapeutic interventions. *Ageing Res. Rev.* 2006, 5(4): 449–67. Epub 2006 Sep 11.

105. Grønbaek, K.; Treppendahl, M.; Asmar, F.; Guldberg, P. Epigenetic changes in cancer as potential targets for prophylaxis and maintenance therapy. *Basic Clin Pharmacol. toxicol.* 2008, 103(5):389–96. doi: 10.1111/j.1742 -7843.2008.00325.x.

106. Nasef A.; Chapel, A.; Mazurier, C.; Bouchet, S.; Lopez, M.; Mathieu, N.; Sensebé, L.; Zhang, Y.; Gorin, N.C.; Thierry, D.; et al. Identification of IL-10 and TGF-beta transcripts involved in the inhibition of T-lymphocyte prolif-eration during cell contact with human mesenchymal stem cells. *Gene Expr.* 2007, 3: 217–226.

107. Ryan, J. M.; Barry, F.; Murphy, J. M.; Mahon, B. P. Interferon-gamma does not break, but promotes the immunosuppressive capacity of adult human mesen-chymal stem cells. *Clin Exp Immunol.* 2007, 149: 353–363.

108. Ortiz, L. A.; Dutreil, M.; Fattman, C.; Pandey, A. C.; Torres, G.; Go, K.; Phinney, D. G. Interleukin 1 receptor antagonist mediates the antiinflamma-tory and antifibrotic effect of mesenchymal stem cells during lung injury. *Proc Natl Acad Sci USA* 2007, 104: 11002–11007.

109. English, K.; Barry, F. P.; Field-Corbett, C. P.; Mahon, B. P. IFN-gamma and TNF-alpha differentially regulate immunomodulation by murine mesenchymal stem cells. *Immunol Lett.* 2007, 110: 91–100.

110. Augello, A.; Tasso, R.; Negrini, S. M.; Cancedda, R.; Pennesi G. Cell therapy using allogeneic bone marrow mesenchymal stem cells prevents tissue damage in collagen-induced arthritis. *Arthritis Rheum* 2007, 56 :1175–1186.

111. Parekkadan, B.; Tilles, A. W.; Yarmush, M. L. Bone marrow-derived mesen-chymal stem cells ameliorate autoimmune enteropathy independently of regu-latory T cells. *Stem Cells* 2008, 26: 1913–1919.

112. Hanley E. N., Jr. Human adipose-derived mesenchymal stem cells: serial passaging, doubling time and cell senescence. *Biotech Histochem* 2012, 87: 303–311.

113. Han, S. M.; Han, S. H.; Coh, Y. R.; Jang, G.; Chan, R. J.; Kang, S. K.; Lee, H. W.; Youn H. Y. Enhanced proliferation and differentiation of Oct4- and Sox2-overexpressing human adipose tissue mesenchymal stem cells. *Exp Mol Med* 2014, 46: e101.

114. Biava, P. M.; Bonsignorio, D.; Hoxa, M. Cell proliferation curves of different human tumor lines after in vitro treatment with Zebrafish embryonic extracts. *J. Tumor Marker Oncol.*, 2001, 16 195–202.

115. Biava, P. M.; Carluccio, A. Activation of anti-oncogene p53 produced by embryonic extracts in vitro tumor cells. *J. Tumor Marker Oncol.*, 1977, 12, 9–15.

116. Biava, P. M.; Bonsignorio, D.; Hoxa, M.; Facco, R.; Ielapi, T.; Frati, L.; Bizzarri, M. Post-traslational modification of the retinoblastoma protein (pRb) induced by in vitro administration of Zebrafish embryonic extracts on human kidney adenocarcinoma cell line. *J. Tumor Marker Oncol.*, 2002, 17(2); 59–64.

117. Biava P. M, Monguzzi A, Bonsignorio D, Frosi A, Sell S, Klavins JV. Xenopus Laevis Embryos share antigens with Zebrafish Embryos and with human malignant neoplasms *J. Tumor Marker Oncol.* 2001, 16; 203–206.

118. Biava, P. M.; Bonsignorio, D. Cancer and cell differentiation: a model to explain malignancy. *J. Tumor Marker Oncol.* 2002, 17(3): 47–54.

119. Cucina, A.; Biava, P. M.; D'Anselmi, F.; Coluccia, P.; Conti, F.; Di Clemente, R.; Miccheli, A.; Frati, L.; Gulino, A.; Bizzarri, M. Zebrafish embryo proteins induce apoptosis in human colon cancer cells (Caco2). *Apoptosis,* 2006, 9, 1617–1628.

120. D'Anselmi F, Cucina A, Biava PM, Proietti S, Coluccia P, Frati L, Bizzarri M. (2011) Zebrafish stem cell differentiation stage factors suppress Bcl-xL release and enhance 5 Fu mediated apoptosis in colon cancer cells. *Curr Pharm Biotechnol* 2011, 12: 261–267.

121. Biava P.M., Nicolini A., Ferrari P., Sell S. A systemic approach to cancer treatment: tumor cell reprogramming focused on endocrine-related cancers. *Curr. Med. Chem.* 2014, 9: 1072–1081.

122. Livraghi, T.; Meloni, F.; Frosi, A.; Lazzaroni, S.; Bizzarri, M.; Frati, L.; Biava, P.M. Treatment with stem cell differentiation stage factors of intermediate-advanced hepatocellular carcinoma: an open randomized clinical trial. *Oncol Res.,* 2005, 15 (7,8): 399–408.

123. Livraghi T, Ceriani R, Palmisano A, Pedicini V, Pich MG, Tommasini MA, Torzilli G. Complete response in 5 out of 38 patients with advanced

hepatocellular carcinoma treated with stem cell differentiation stage factors: case reports from a single centre. *Curr Pharm Biotechnol* 2011, 12: 254–260.

124. Norata G,; Biava P.. M.; Di Pierro F. The Zebrafish embryo derivative affects cell viability of epidermal cells: a possible role in the treatment of psoriasis. Giornale Ital. *Dermatol. Venereol.* 2013, 148 (5):479–483.

125. Canaider, S.; Maioli, M.; Facchin, F.; Bianconi, E.; Santaniello, S.; Pigliaru, G.; Ljungberg, L.; Burigana, F; Bianchi, F.; Olivi, E.; Tremolada, C.; Biava, P. M.; Ventura, C. Human stem cell exposure to developmental stage zebrafish extracts: a novel strategy for tuning stemness and senescence patterning. *CellR4,* 2014, 2(5), 1226.

126. Lunde K, Belting H. G, Driever W. Zebrafish pou5f1/pou2, homolog of mammalian Oct4, functions in the endoderm specification cascade. *Curr Biol* 2004; 14: 48–55.

127. Onichtchouk D, Geier F, Polok B, Messerschmidt D. M, Mössner R, Wendik B, Song S, Taylor V, Timmer J, Driever W. Zebrafish Pou5f1-dependent transcriptional networks in temporal control of early development. *Mol Syst Biol* 2010; 6: 354.

128. Kotkamp K, Mössner R, Allen A, Onichtchouk D, Driever W. A Pou5f1/Oct4 dependent Klf2a, Klf2b, and Klf17 regulatory sub-network contributes to EVL and ectoderm development during zebrafish embryogenesis. *Dev Biol* 2014; 385: 433–447.

129. Campisi J, Dimri G. P. Control of the replicative life span of human fibroblasts by p16 and the polycomb protein Bmi-1. *Mol Cell Biol* 2003; 23: 389–401.

130. Klapper W, Parwaresch R, Krupp G. Telomere biology in human aging and aging syndromes. *Mech Ageing Dev* 2001; 122: 695–712.

131. Wilsker D, Patsialou A, Dallas PB, Moran E. ARID proteins: A diverse family of DNA binding proteins implicated in the control of cell growth, differentiation, and development. *Cell Growth Differ* 2002; 13: 95–106.

132. Popowski M, Templeton TD, Lee BK, Rhee C, Li H, Miner C, Dekker JD, Orlanski S, Bergman Y, Iyer VR, Webb CF, Tucker H. Bright/Arid3A acts as a barrier to somatic cell reprogramming through direct regulation of Oct4, Sox2, and Nanog. *Stem Cell Reports* 2014; 2: 26–35.

133. Barakat MT, Humke EW, Scott MP. Learning from Jekyll to control Hyde: Hedgehog signaling in development and cancer. *Trends Mol. Med* 2010, 16(8): 337–348.

Cancer: A Problem of Developmental Biology. The Scientific Evidence for Reprogramming and Differentiation Therapy

Current Drug Targets, 2016, Volume 17, Number 10:1103–10.
© Bentham Science Publishers.

S. Sell, A. Nicolini, P. Ferrari, P. M. Biava

This article begins with research undertaken in the late seventies that led some researchers to interpret cancer as being due to the presence of embryonic cells blocked in their process of maturation (maturation arrest). It reviews the theory of maturation arrest in the light of recent research on the epigenetic code and its ability to regulate gene expression. Tumor diseases on the basis of more recent research are interpreted as being due to genetic and/or epigenetic alterations that require reprogramming. The article reviews the important reprogramming and differentiation treatments of cancer cells and concludes that tumor diseases are pathologies of stem-cell development and not simply due to maturation arrest. They were caused by many modifications and require treatment by epigenetic reprogramming.

Introduction

In 1978, B. Pierce and colleagues published a book entitled *Cancer: A Problem of Developmental Biology*.[1] Based on their work on embryonal carcinoma, Pierce and colleagues predicted the present concept of tissue determined stem cells[2] in which tissue renewal is accomplished by asymmetric division of a stem cell to produce one daughter cell that remains a stem cell and a second daughter cell that becomes a proliferation of transit amplifying cells. The progeny of the transit amplifying cells eventually terminally differentiate into mature cells. According to this model, the main difference between normal tissue renewal and proliferation of cancer cells is that the transit amplifying cells of the cancer do not terminally differentiate as do normal transit amplifying cells, but continue to proliferate. However, Pierce and

Wallace[3] found that even the proliferating progeny of "stem" cells of a squamous cell carcinoma could give rise to daughter cells that differentiate into mature keratinized cells. In normal tissue renewal, there is equilibrium between the rate of proliferation and the rate of cell death so that the number of cells at any given time is relatively constant. In contrast, in cancer tissue the equilibrium is shifted in favor of proliferation over cell loss so that in cancers the number of cells continues to increase. The key concept is that cancers are maintained by cancer stem cells that give rise to daughter transit amplifying cells that do not mature at a normal rate and continue to increase in number. This is known as maturation arrest.[4]

An even earlier model of cancer based on an origin from stem cells was the embryonal rest theory of cancer.[5] The first theory of the origin of cancer was a "field theory." Field theories are based on the idea that the tissues surrounding the cells at risk (niche) provide a signal or environment that acts to stimulate the cells to proliferate as cancer cells.[5-6] The first idea that cancers might arise from stem cells appeared in the early 19th century.[7-8] Although the concept of stem cells was still far in the future, Durante[9] and Conheim[10] introduced the idea that cancers arise from embryonal tissue that survived in adult organs; i.e., embryonal rests. They proposed that disequilibrium between the embryonal cells in the "rest" and the surrounding tissue allowed these remnants of embryonic tissue to reassume proliferation and produce masses of cells that resembled fetal tissues. This mechanism of cancer development is consistent with a field theory; i.e., a change in the tissue stroma allows cancer to appear but also identifies the cells of origin as stem cells. However, by the early 1900s the embryonic rest theory lost support,[6] and in general, interest in cancer research waned as the primary focus for research and clinical studies was infectious diseases. It would take 50 more years before studies on teratocarcinoma would lead to a reassertion of the embryonic rest theory of cancer in the form of the stem-cell theory of cancer.

Teratocarcinoma

Teratocarcinomas consist of mature, differentiated tissues, as well as fetal components: yolk sac and placental elements. The production of alphafetoprotein (AFP) by the yolk sac component and of human chorionic gonadotropin (hCG) by the placental elements suggests that the embryonal cells of a teratocarcinoma are totipotent; i.e., they can differentiate into both adult and embryonic cells. The growth of these tumors may be followed by measuring the serum levels of AFP or hCG. Most of the cells of a teratocarcinoma are mature and non-malignant; the malignant cells are located in the embryo's body, a tissue structure that contains undifferentiated embryo tissue. The cancer stem-cell nature of these cells is documented by their ability to form cancers upon transplantation into histocompatible recipients. The normal stem-cell properties of these cells are demonstrated by the fact that transplantation into the inner cell mass of a developing blastocyst results in incorporation of teratocarcinoma, the cells into normal developing tissues.[11-16] Convincing documentation of the tissue stem-cell origin of cancer was obtained in the 1960s, when Leroy Stevens was able to produce growth of malignant teratocarcinomas after transplanting normal germinal stem cells from the genital ridge of day 12 SIJ/129 male mice into the testicles of normal 129 adult male mice. In the testicular transplant niche the germinal stem cells grew abnormally and formed tumors, thus supporting both the stem-cell origin of the cancer and the field theory of cancer.[17-18] Then about a decade later it was demonstrated that teratocarcinoma cells did not grow when transplanted into a mouse blastocyst. The cells from these transplantable teratocarcinomas injected into normal blastocysts became incorporated into the developing embryos. The resulting adult mice had organs that were made up of a mixture of mature tissues from the normal blastocyst and from the cancer (Chimera). The inner cell mass of the blastocyst is able to reprogram both mature tissue stem cells as well as cancer stem cells.[19-25] Thus, a combined stem-cell field theory of cancer is supported by the observation that teratocarcinomas arise from tissue germinal stem cells if the cells are placed in an environment that allows expression of the malignant phenotype.

Barry Pierce and his co-workers extensively examined the cellular make up of teratocarcinomas.[1,25] From their studies Pierce hypothesized a hierarchical model of cancer, with cancer stem cells giving rise to cancer transit amplifying cells that would exhibit various stages of differentiation culminating in terminally differentiated cells, and this hierarchical model was extended to provide a general thesis for the cells that make up any cancer.[1] They postulated that the differentiation state of a cancer depends upon the stage of maturation at which the majority of cells of the cancer become arrested. If maturation arrest occurs at an early stage the tumor will be poorly differentiated and most of the tumor transit amplifying cells will be able to divide; if at a later stage, the tumor will be well differentiated and few of the tumor transit amplifying cells will divide. In either case, the tumor will be maintained by cancer stem cells that provide the self renewing cells of the tumor.

Control of Differentiation by
the Embryo's Microenvironment

The tissues of the embryo are able to induce differentiation of normal and cancer stem cells,[26-27] including putative carcinogen induced cancer cells. Exposure of developing embryos to chemical carcinogens may lead to malformations, but not to cancer. Thus, the embryonic microenvironment is able to correct for the mutations induced by carcinogens and prevent cancer formation.[28-29] As stated above, the blastocyst environment also controls growth of transplanted malignant cells, whereas malignant cells placed in other sites of the developing embryo, such as the perivitelline space, are not controlled.[30-32] On the other hand, more differentiated tissues of the embryo may also regulate growth of cancer cells that are normally found in that tissue. There is also evidence for diffusible factors produced by blastocyst cells that may induce differentiation of cancer stem cells. The regulatory environment of the blastocyst is not limited to teratocarcinoma. Other cancers shown to be converted to normal developing tissue when placed in an appropriate embryonic microenvironment include leukemia, melanoma, hepatocellular cancer and breast cancer.[33-37] Malignant melanoma cells placed into the extraembryonal membrane of the Zebrafish differentiated into normal neural crest like cells.[38] Thus, different embryonal microenvironments may have different differentiation potentials related to normal cellular differentiation. For example, the placenta may also regulate transplanted leukemia cells.[39] Other authors obtained similar results with different experiments[40-41] and concluded that embryomother cross-talk is very important in determining the arrest of tumor growth, because both maternal (decidua) and embryonic tissues contain substances with anti-cancer properties, which cooperate, inhibiting or delaying tumor growth.[40] These promising results open new perspectives not only in cancer biology comprehension, but also in leading to a different therapeutic strategy. In fact in the last years many studies have clarified that embryonic cells share fundamental features with tumor cells,[42-43] such as proliferation and expression of embryonic proteins (AFP, or ABC transporters), common molecular signals and pathways (i.e., beta-catenin/TCF/WNT Notch, BMP and Hedgehog signals),[44-46] anaerobic metabolism,[47] etc. In addition, epithelial-to-mesenchymal transition (EMT) observed in cancer tissue[48-49] may also be viewed as a "reactivation" of an embryonic program.[50-51]

These findings illustrate that cancer is a disease of developmental biology. To understand how the substances taken from developing embryo or other biological substances are able to induce differentiation of cancer cells, we are here reporting important results on reprogramming and differentiation treatment.

Reprogramming and Differentiation
Treatment of Cancer Cells

The term "cancer cell reprogramming" is used to define any kind of intervention aimed at transforming cancer cells into terminally differentiated cells. Differentiation treatments have the same goal; that is, to induce terminal differentiation of cancer cells or to force cancer stem cells to become transit amplifying cells that can then be treated by additional treatment such as chemotherapy or radiation. This review reports on advances of these technologies, including our personal contributions. An example of one of the first applications of differentiation therapy is the removal of the block to differentiation in human myeloid leukemia.[52-53] The genetic lesions of leukemia result in a block of differentiation (maturation arrest) that allows myeloid leukemic cells to continue to proliferate and/or prevents the terminal differentiation and apoptosis seen in normal white blood cells. In chronic myeloid leukemia, the bcr-abl (t9/22) translocation produces a fusion product that is an activated tyrosine kinase resulting in constitutive activation cells at the myelocyte level. This activation may be inhibited by imatinib mesylate (Gleevec, STI-571), which blocks the binding of ATP to the activated tyrosine kinase, prevents phosphorylation, and allows the leukemic cells to differentiate and undergo apoptosis. In acute promyelocytic leukemia, fusion of the retinoic acid receptor-alpha with the gene coding for promyelocytic protein, the PML-RAR alpha (t15:17) translocation, produces a fusion product that blocks the activity of the promyelocytic protein, which is required for the formation of the granules of promyelocytes and prevents further differentiation. Retinoic acids (RA) bind to the retinoic acid receptor (RAR alpha) component of the fusion product, resulting in degradation of the fusion protein by ubiquitinization. This allows normal PML to participate in granule formation and differentiation of the promyelocytes.

Unfortunately, there are cases of RA resistance. This is a serious problem for patients with acute promyelocytic leukemia who are receiving all-trans retinoic acids. The biologic effects of RA are mediated by two distinct families of transcriptional factors: RA receptors (RARs) and retinoid X receptors (RXRs). RXRs heterodimerize with 1, 25-dihydroxyvitamin D3 [1,25(OH)2D3] receptor (VDR), enabling their efficient transcriptional activation. The cyclin-dependent kinase (cdk) inhibitor p21(WAF1/CIP1) has a vitamin D3–responsive element (VDRE) in its promoter, and 1,25(OH)2D3 enhances the expression of p21(WAF1/CIP1) and induces differentiation of leukemic cell lines. In this case 1,25(OH)2D3 induces increased expression of cdk inhibitors, which mediates a G1 arrest, and this may be associated with differentiation of RA-resistant cells toward mature granulocytes.[54] In addiction it is here recorded that the vitamin D anti-tumor effects are inhibited by CYP24A1 gene, which encodes 24-Hydrolase, the key enzyme for degrading many forms of vitamin D, including the most active form 1,25D(3). The inhibition of CYP24A1 by 4,5,6,7 tetrabromobenzimidazole (TBBZ) in human prostate cancer enhances 1,25D(3) mediated anti-tumor effect.[55] It is here also recorded that curcumin, a bioactive polyphenol found in curry and several of its analogs, elicits transcriptional activation in retinoic acid and retinoid X receptor (RXR) responsive systems and stimulates RXR homodimerization and vitamin D receptor (VDR)–coactivator interaction.[56] Finally, retinoid and their receptors play an important role in controlling the progression of many other tumors.[57]

The Use of Stem Cell Differentiation Stage Factors (SCDFs)

The application of stem cell differentiation stage factors (SCDFs) to revert cancer cells into a benign phenotype was started many years ago. SCDFs in the form of factors taken from Zebrafish embryos at different stages of development demonstrated a significant inhibition of proliferation of different human tumor lines in vitro (glioblastoma multiforme, melanoma, hepatocellular carcinoma, breast carcinoma, kidney adenocarcinoma, colon adenocarcinoma, acute lymphoblastic leukemia).[58] The molecules that play a key role in the regulation process of the cell cycle, such as p53[59] and pRb,[60] are involved through transcriptional and post-translational processes. In addition, treatment of colon cancer with SCDSFs induces caspase 3 activation, mainly by increasing the release of E2F-1, leading to c-Myc overexpression and the activation of a p73 apoptotic-dependent pathway.

There is also a concurrent significant normalization of the ratio of e-cadherin to beta catenin, with an increase in e-cadherin levels.[61] Finally, SCDSFs induce an almost complete growth inhibition of cell proliferation of CaCo2 colon cancer cell line after the concurrent treatment with 5 Fluorouracil,[62] suggesting that Zebrafish embryo factors improve chemotherapy efficacy with 5 Fluorouracil. Subcutaneous injection of SCDFs with primary Lewis Lung Carcinoma cells into C57BL/6 female syngeneic mice produces a highly significant difference (P<0.001) between treated and control mice, both in terms of primary tumor growth and survival compared to untreated controls.[63] A randomized clinical trial that was conducted between January 1, 2001, and April 30, 2004, on 179 patients with intermediate-advanced hepatocellular carcinoma unresponsive to conventional treatment (transplantation, resection, ablation therapy, or chemoembolization). The patients were treated with a product developed following the aforementioned in vitro and in vivo studies. It contained SCDSFs taken from Zebrafish embryos at a very low concentration (micrograms). This was administered sublingually at a dose of 30 drops to the patients three times a day. Regression occurred in 19.8% of the patients (2.4% of complete regression and 17.4% of partial regression) and 16% disease stabilization, with over 60% survival rate after 40 months in the patients who responded to treatment, compared to 10% in the remaining patients. The performance status improved in 82.6% of the treated patients, including those in advanced stages of the disease.[64]

Another clinical trial was conducted on 50 patients with "advanced" stage HCC from 2005 to 2010. Complete response was regarded as sustained disappearance of the neoplastic lesions, accompanied by normalization of AFP levels. In 13.1% of the patients with "advanced" stage there was a sustained complete response. No side effects occurred.[65] This favorable result using SCDSFs therapy of patients with "advanced" HCC encouraged further testing of other reprogramming treatment.

Other Reprogramming Treatments
Oocyte Extracts
Extracts taken from prophase amphibian oocytes of axolotl (AOE) and xenopus (XOE) induce re-expression of some tumor suppressor genes. RARB, CST6, CCND2, GAS2 and CDKN2A are silenced or expressed at very low levels in MCF-7 and HCC 1954 cell lines representing luminal and basal breast cancer phenotypes.[66] Extracts of AOE and XOE prophase oocytes induce re-expression of these genes in both breast cancer cell lines.

Naive Human Umbilical Cord Matrix Derived Stem Cells
Human umbilical cord matrix stem cells (hUCMSCs) are unique stem cells derived from Warton's jelly (termed Warton's jelly stromal cells).[67] Metastatic growth of MDA-231 human breast carcinoma cells is attenuated in culture and in a mouse xenograft experimental model by un-engineered (naive) human umbilical cord matrix stem cells (hUCMSC).[68] In vitro, culture of hUCMSC with MDA-231 carcinoma cells inhibits DNA synthesis, increases the G2 cell population and inhibits colony growth of the carcinoma cells. The inhibited growth of cancer cells appears to be due to blocking of ERK-1/2 and PI3K/Akt signaling with activation of intrinsic apoptosis signals.

Reprogramming Telomerase and the MAT-8 Gene
A subpopulation of cancer stem-like cells in prostate cancer cell lines and primary prostate cancer tissues that are highly tumorigenic expresses some essential stem-cell-associated transcription factors (Oct3/4, Sox2, Nanog, Klf4, and c-myc).[69] Due to their importance in prostate cancer growth, these cancer stem cells seem a likely target for novel strategies for prostate cancer therapy. One of these novel strategies is related to the enzyme telomerase. Malignant cells from many cancers have significant

telomerase expression and activity levels that correlate directly with malignant metastatic potential. New gene constructs to reprogram telomerase have been engineered and validated: 1) small interfering RNA against wild type mouse telomerase RNA (alpha MTer-siRNA); 2) mutant-template mouse telomerase RNA (MT-mTer), which encodes incorrect mouse telomeric repeats.

Lentiviral delivery of alpha mTer-siRNA to mouse prostate cancer cells caused growth inhibition and rapid apoptosis in cancer progenitor cells isolated from human prostatectomy specimens.[70-71] Transfection of human PC-3 and LNCaP prostate carcinoma cells with small interfering double-stranded RNA (siRNA) oligonucleotides against the MAT-8 gene produced a specific down-regulation of MAT-8 expression and a significant decrease in cellular proliferation of both cancer cell lines.[72]

Artificial Transcription Factors (ATFs) in Breast Cancer Cells

The epigenetic reprogramming of breast cancer cells may be accomplished by targeted DNA methylation.[73] Site specific DNA methylation and prolonged stable repression of the tumor suppressor Maspin and the oncogene Sox2 can be obtained in breast cancer cells by Zinc-finger ATFs targeting DNA methyltransferase-3a to the promoters of these genes.

Stimulation of Immunity to Cancer By
Reprogramming Tumor-Associated Dendritic Cells

The endocytic activity and immune activation of ovarian cancer-associated dendritic cells (DC) may be selectively increased by treatment with the immunostimulatory miRNA miR-155. Nanoparticles carrying oligonucleotide duplexes mimicking the bulged structure of endogenous pre-miRNA strongly enhanced miR-155 activity without saturating the RNA-induced silencing complex that produced genome-wide transcriptional changes that in turn silenced multiple immunosuppressive mediators. Tumor infiltrating DCs were transformed from immunosuppressive to highly immunostimulatory cells, activating strong antitumor responses that impeded the progression of established ovarian cancer.[74]

Also the transfer of chromosome 3p fragments in a novel epithelial ovarian cancer cell line model (OV-90) induces tumor suppression. Tumor suppression is associated with a modified transcriptome by microarray analysis. Reprogramming of the transcriptome appears to be a consequence of the chromosome 3 transfer and tumor suppression affected molecular networks sustaining ovarian carcinogenesis.[75]

Discussion

The use of SCDSFs in anti-tumor treatment has led to a cancer model[76] that is consistent with the scientific and clinical evidence. This model integrates that of Pierce and collaborators and views cancer as a consequence of two different processes: 1) maturation arrest and 2) a stochastic process in which genetic and epigenetic alterations conduce a normal differentiated cell to be malignant. These two process are not mutually exclusive, and both have been invoked.[77-79] The process of maturation arrest has already been described in this review. In the stochastic process the initial mechanism could be a mutation or an epigenetic alteration. If the process begins with a mutation, the minimal number of stochastic mutational events which can transform a normal cell in a cancer cell is calculated between four and seven.[80] If mutations are introduced into normal cells in a non-stochastic manner, i.e., triggering at precise genes, the number is reduced.[81] The preferred targets of these mutations are genes encoding for key-role effectors of cell cycle regulation and cell signaling, and for growth factors and their receptors. Mutations are either gain-of-function, in the case of proto-oncogenes, or loss-of-function, in the case of tumor-suppressor genes.

Nevertheless, defining the transformation of a normal cell into a cancer cell as the result of a sum of mutations may be reductionistic. For normal cells to become cancerous, transformation also depends on a complex network of surrounding microenvironmental signals from cell-to-cell "cross-talking" or from soluble extracellular factors. For example, it is well known that inflammatory cells sustain rather than fight tumor growth[82] and that pro-inflammatory cytokines promote cancer cell proliferation by inhibiting tumor-suppression pathways.[83] The whole context is thus critical in terms of determining cell fate in line with a complex view of cell biology.[84] According to this view, cancer could be defined as a microevolutive process that is usually the consequence of a high variability of the mechanisms used by cells to become malignant. Nonetheless the model of cancer described by one of us[76] assumes that regardless of how the steps in these genetic pathways are arranged, development of all types of tumor is governed by a final common process. Some authors define "early crisis" and "genetic catastrophe" of cells as steps enabling the evolving population of premalignant cells to reach malignancy. As a result of these crises a cell has two possibilities after each crisis: either die or survive.

In other words, surviving cells begin a chaotic process with a series of multiple bifurcations, at the end of which cells become cancerous. The research we have carried out has shown that the chaotic process is stabilized by what chaos theory refers to as an "attractor," which leads the tumor cell genome to a new configuration. In other words, the process which causes cancer is a process of deterministic chaos.

Cancer Stem-like Cells

Depending on the degree of malignancy, the cancer cell configuration is similar to that present in stem cells at various stages of development and differentiation. Our experiments have shown that tumor cells are undifferentiated cells, blocked in a multiplication phase between two cell differentiation stages. Tumor cells can therefore be considered as cells in which both genetic and epigenetic changes are usually present, these last changes being linked to the new gene configurations, very similar to those present in stem cells. The above process describes the mechanisms that can transform a normal differentiated cell into a cancer cell, but the mechanisms of carcinogenesis can from the outset concern the normal stem cells present in a specific tissue. In this latter case, the process is simpler but the result is the same: the transformation of a normal cell into a cancer stem-like cell. In this case, the model of Pierce and collaborators (maturation arrest) is sufficient to explain the origin of cancer, while the transformation of a complete differentiated cell in cancer cell requires a stochastic model of deterministic chaos to explain the process. The model cited in this article,[76] conceived in 2002, describes both the processes that give rise to all kinds of cancer. In this model the most aggressive tumors are those with genetic configurations present in the early stages of embryonic differentiation, while the well-differentiated tumor cells are those present in the final stages of cell differentiation. The current classifications of tumors are redundant because they do not consider that from an ontogenetic viewpoint, as a cancer that originates in a specific organ becomes increasingly aggressive and flows into cell types that share the same genetic configuration with cancers of other organs.

Finally, some tumor types are made up of differing cellular clones with varying degrees of malignancy and thus of cells with genetic configurations that derive from various stages of differentiation. So this model of cancer is consistent with the real situation and has been supported by our experiments. They demonstrate that the factors differentiating stem cells are capable of differentiating even tumor cells or causing their apoptosis, by-passing the mutations or correcting the epigenetic alterations that are at the origin of malignancy. In line with this approach, we recall the characteristics shared by both tumor and normal stem cells: tumor cells have oncofetal antigens, which are maintained during phylogenesis,[85] and specific receptors on the cell membrane on which stem cell differentiation factors likely act. In addition, tumor and stem cells have common signals and pathways such as APC/beta-catenin/TCF/Wnt pathways, and Hedgehog/Smoothened/Patched pathways, as already described.

The problem with tumor cells is twofold: not only do they harbor genetic mutations, which usually underlie the malignancy, but they also have significant modifications of the epigenetic code. The genetic configuration and metabolism of tumor cells are very similar to those of stem cells in that both have active proto-oncogenes; both produce embryonic growth factors; both, as already mentioned, have oncofetal antigens; and both function with an anaerobic metabolism. The difference between stem and tumor cells lies in the fact that the latter can no longer complete development and differentiate, in view of the mutations. The use of SCDSFs results in tumor cells falling within the scope of normal physiology, blocking the cell cycle and activating metabolic pathways of differentiation or apoptosis. In this way, the mutations—and hence the malignancy—can be by-passed.

In recent years, some studies have linked a tumor's malignancy and chemoresistance to the presence of cancer stem cells,[85] which are responsible for the repopulation of a tumor after chemotherapy.[86] Cancer stem-like cells have been identified in various solid tumors, such as glioblastoma multiforme,[87-89] breast cancer,[90-93] lung cancer,[94-97] prostate cancer,[98-100] ovarian cancer,[101-104] liver cancer,[105-109] gastric cancer,[110-115] colon cancer,[116-118] pancreas cancer,[119-121] and squamous carcinoma of the head and neck,[122-125] etc. Moreover, the presence of cancer stem cells has long been known to be characteristic of many hematological malignant diseases.

Conclusions

Ongoing studies are providing important clarification of the different mechanisms of cell differentiation and the various metabolic pathways common to cancer and stem cells. One example is the research carried out at the Children's Memorial Hospital in Chicago. As mentioned, these studies have confirmed that a malignant melanoma reverts to a normal phenotype when exposed to the microenvironment of the Zebrafish embryo. This occurs because a central nervous system morphogen (called Nodal and a member of the TGF-beta superfamily)—

which is re-expressed in the cells of the malignant melanoma and responsible for the melanoma's aggressiveness—is downregulated by a factor present in an embryonic environment; for example, Lefty.[126] This approach falls within the differentiation and reprogramming therapy concept that researchers have for some time hoped to pursue and that wholly supports our studies. The proposed model of cancer[76] takes account of the necessary complexity of reprogramming treatments. In fact, cell differentiation mechanisms consist of a multigenic regulation, so that a more differentiated cell differs from a less differentiated one because of the change in expression of a large number of genes.

If the ultimate goal is the differentiation rather than destruction of the cancer cell, this can clearly be achieved only by providing the cell with all the factors that are necessary for reprogramming. These can all be found when life is forming. In fact, during organogenesis the entire repertoire of regulatory molecules able to differentiate stem cells is present (transcriptional, post-transcriptional, translational, post-translational regulatory factors). Each kind of cancer stem cell can revert to a normal phenotype only when the regulation network of differentiation is specific and complete enough for that kind of cancer cell. As a result, focus should be on microenvironment and networks of the biological structures, rather than on individual, specific mechanisms. This does not mean that research into molecular mechanisms should be disregarded. In fact, any new elucidated molecular pathway illuminates one more piece of the puzzle. Indeed, the difficulty in bridging the gap to a new scientific paradigm, i.e., shifting our view from reductionism to complexity, has been the main barrier to acquiring a more complete knowledge of cancer.

Research on stem-cell differentiation and other work based on a more extended approach to cancer treatment together yield a more complete understanding of the biological processes that sustain tumor growth. These studies are in progress worldwide and the scientific community is now ready to accept the new paradigm, as a number

Cancer: A Problem of Developmental Biology; Scientific Evidence for Reprogramming and Differentiation Therapy

1) Many experiments demonstrated that cancer can be considered a deviation in normal development, which can be regulated by factors of the embryonic microenvironment.

2) The most important researches about the reprogramming and differentiation treatments of cancer cells are recorded in the article.

3) A model of cancer that integrates the theory of the "maturation arrest" with the theory that describes cancer as a process of deterministic chaos determined by genetic or epigenetic alterations in differentiated cells is here proposed (Fig. 1 Biava 2002).

4) The researches described in the article demonstrated that cancer can be considered a problem of developmental biology and that one of the most important hallmarks of cancer is the loss of differentiation.

Fig. 1 CANCER AS A PROCESS OF DETERMINISTIC CHAOS - Legend
<u>A</u>: normal cell   <u>B</u>: cell with damaged DNA   <u>C</u>: cell with rampant genetic instability
<u>D</u>: cancer cell: stable gene configuration with uncoupled steps of cell multiplication and differentiation
<u>E</u>: stem cell   <u>F</u>: committed stem cell   <u>G</u>: differentiating cell   <u>H</u>: differentiated cell

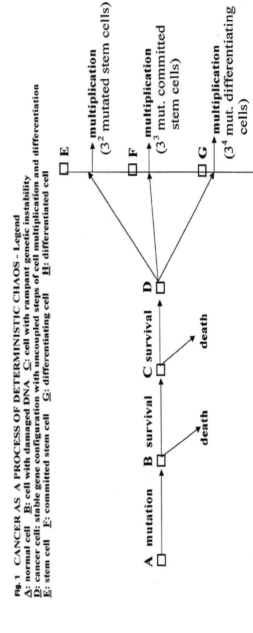

of authors confirm.[127] In this vision it was proposed in a recent review[128] a new hallmark of cancer: the loss of differentiation of the cancer cell. This confirms that cancer is a problem of developmental biology.

References

1. Pierce GB, Shikes R, Fink LM. *Cancer: a problem of developmental biology.* Englewood Cliffs, New Jersey; Prentice Hall Inc, 197.

2. Pierce GB, Spears WC. Tumors as caricatures of the process of tissue renewal: prospects for therapy by directing differentiation. *Cancer Res* 1988; 48: 1196–204.

3. Pierce BB, Wallace C. Differentiation of malignant to benign cells. *Cancer Res* 1971; 31: 127–34.

4. Sell S, Pierce GB. Biology of disease: Maturation arrest of stem cell differentiation is a common pathway for the cellular origin of teratocarcinomas and epithelial cancers. *Lab. Invest* 1994;70: 6–21.

5. Shimkin M. Contrary to Nature. NIH, USDOH, 1977.

6. Bainbridge WS. *The Cancer Problem,* The Macmillan Co. New York, 1914.

7. Recamier JCA. *Recherches sur le traitement du cancer: par la compression methodique simple ou combinee, et sur l'histoire general de la meme maladie.* Paris Gabon 1829.

8. Remak R. Ein beitrag zur entwickelungsgeschichte der krebshaften geschwulste. *Deut Klin* 1854;6: 170–74.

9. Durante F. Nesso fisio-pathologico tra la struttura dei nei materni e la genesi di alcuni tumori maligni. *Arch Memorie ed Osservazioni di Chirugia Pratica* 1874; 11: 217–26.

10. Cohnheim J. Congenitales, quergestreiftes muskelsarkon der nireren. *Virchows Arch* 1875; 65: 64.

11. Osler W, McCrea T. *Modern Medicine: It's Theory and Practice.* Lea and Ferbiger, Philadelphia and New York, 1913.

12. Dixon FJ, Moore RA. Testicular tumors: a clinicopathological study. *Cancer* 1953; 6: 417–43.

13. Damjanov I. Pathobiology of human germ cell tumors. Recent Results *Cancer Research* 1991; 123: 1–34.

14. Solter D, Damjanov I. Teratocarcinoma and the expression of ondo-developmental genes. *Methods Cancer Res* 1979; 18: 277–98.

15. Chan D, Sell S. Tumor Markers. In: *Teitz Textbook of Clinical Chemistry;* Burtis CA, Ashwood ER Eds. Philadelphia, PA: Saunders 1999, pp 722–49.

16. Peyron A. Sur la presence des cellules genitales primordiales dans les boutons embryononnaires des embryomes parthenogenetiques chez lhomme. *Cr R Acad Sci* (Paris) 1938: 206: 1680–83.

17. Stevens LC. Experimental production of testicular teratomas in mice. *Proc Natl Acad Sci USA* 1964;52: 654–61.

18. Stevens LC. Origin of testicular teratomas from primordial germ cells in mice. *J Natl Cancer Inst* 1967;38: 549–52.

19. Brinster RL. The effect of cells transferred into the mouse blastocyst on subsequent development. *J Exp Med* 1974:140: 1049–56.

20. Mintz B, Illmensee K. Normal genetically mosaic mice produced from malignant teratocarcinoma cells. *Proc Natl Acad Sci USA* 1975; 72: 3583–9.

21. Ilmmenesee K. Reversion of malignancy and normalized differentiation of teratocarcinoma cells in mammals. In: *Generic mosaics and chimeras in mammals;* Russel LC Editor, New York: Plenum 1978; 3–25.

22. Papaionnou VE, McBurney MW, Gardner RL., Evans RL. Fate of teratocarcinoma cells injected into early mouse embryos. *Nature* 1975; 258: 70–3.

23. Papaioannou VE. Ontogen, pathology, oncology. *Int J Dev Biol* 1993; 37: 33–7.

24. Pierce GB, Dixon FJ. The demonstration of teratogenesis by metamorphosis of multipotential cells. *Cancer* 1959;12: 573–83.

25. Pierce GM, Dixon FJ, Verney E. Teratocarcinogenic and tissue forming potentials of the cell types comprising neoplastic embryoid bodies. *Lab Invest.* 1960;9: 583–602.

26. Brent RL. Radiation Teratogenesis. *Teratology* 1980; 21: 281–98.

27. Einhorm L. Are there factors preventing cancer development during embryonic life? *Oncodev Biol Med* 1982; 4: 219–29.

28. Pierce GB. The cancer cell and its control by the embryo. *Am J Pathol* 1983; 113: 117–24.

29. Pierce GB, Lewis SH, Miller GJ, Morits E, Miller P. Tumorigenicity of embryonal carcinoma as an assay to study control of malignancy by the murine blastocyst. *Proc Natl Acad Sci USA* 1979: 76; 6649–51.

30. Pierce GB, Podesta A, Wells RS. The role of the blastocyst trophoderm in control of colony formation. In: *Teratocarcinoma Stem Cells;* Silver S, Strickland S and Martin G, Eds. New York: Cold Spring Harbor Symposium 1983; pp 15–22.

31. Pierce GB, Pantazis CG, Caldwell JE, Wells RS. Specificity of the control of tumor formation by blastocysts. *Cancer Res* 1982; 1082–7.

32. Gershenson M, Graves K, Carson D, Wells RS, Pierce GB. Regulation of melanoma by the embryonic skin. *Proc Natl Acad Sci USA* 1986:83: 7307–10.

33. Webb CW, Gootwine E, Sachs L. Developmental potential of myeloid leukemia cells injected into rat midgestation embryos. *Dev Biol* 1984; 101: 221–4.

34. Coleman WB, Wennerberg AE, Smith GJ, Grisham JW. Regulation of differentiation of diploid and some aneuploid rat liver epithelial (stemlike) cells by the hepatic microenviromment. *Am J Pathol* 1993;142: 1371–82.

35. Weaver V, Petersen O, Wang F, et al. Reversion of the malignant phenotype of human breast cancer in three-dimensional culture and in vivo by integrin blocking bodies. *J Cell Biol* 1997; 137: 231–45.

36. Postovit LM, Margaryan NV, Seftor EA, et al. Human embryonic stem cell microenvironment suppresses the tumorigenic phenotype of aggressive cancer cells. *Proc Natl Acad Sci USA* 2008; 105: 4329–34.

37. Hendrix MJ, Seftor EA, Seftor REB, et al. Reprogramming metastatic tumor cells with the embryonic microenvironment. *Nat Rev Cancer* 2007; 7: 246–55.

38. Kulesa PM, Kasemeier-Kulesa JC, Teddy JM, et al. Reprogramming metastatic tumor cells to assume a neural crest-like phenotype in an embryonic microenvironment. *Proc Natl Acad Sci USA* 2006; 103: 3752–7.

39. Gootwine E, Webb, CG, Sachs L. Participation of myeloid leukemia cells injected into embryos in haematopoietic differentiation in adult mice. *Nature* 1982; 299: 63–5.

40. Biava PM, Fiorito A, Negro C, Mariani M. Effect of treatment with embryonic and uterine tissue homogenates on Lewis lung carcinoma development. *Cancer Lett* 1988; 41: 265–70.

41. Biava PM, Bonsignorio D, Hoxa M. Life-Protecting Factor (LPF): an anticancer low molecular weight fraction isolated from pregnant uterine mucosa during embryo organogenesis. *J Tumor Marker Oncol* 2000; 15: 223–33.

42. Dalerba P, Cho RW, Clarke MF. Cancer stem cells: models and concepts. *Annu Rev Med* 2007; 58: 267–84.

43. Lee JT, Herlyn M. Embryogenesis meet tumorigenesis. *Nat Med* 2006; 12: 882–3.

44. Katoh M, Katoh M. Transcriptional regulation of WNT2B based on the

balance of Hedgehog, Notch, BMP and WNT signals. *Int J Oncol* 2009; 34: 1411–5.

45. Kathoh M, Katoh M. Transcriptional mechanisms of WNT5A based on NF-kappaB, Hedgehog, TGFbeta, and Notch signaling cascades. *Int J Mol Med* 2009; 23:763–9.

46. Peifer M, Polakis P. WNT signaling in oncogenesis and embryogenesis: a look outside the nucleus. *Science* 2000, 287: 1606–9.

47. Chritofk HF, Vander Heiden MG, Harris MH, et al. The M2 splice isoform of pyruvate kinase is important for cancer metabolism and tumor growth. *Nature* 2008; 452: 230–3.

48. Mani SA, Guo W, Liao M, et al. The epithelial-mesenchymal transition generates cells with properties of stem cells. *Cell* 2008; 133: 704–15.

49. Carro MS, Lim WK, Javier Alvares M, et al. The transcriptional network for mesenchymal transformation of brain tumor. *Nature* 2010; 463: 318–25.

50. Borczuk AC, Gorenstein L, Walter KL, et al. Non small cell lung cancer molecular signature recapitulate lung developmental pathways. *Am J Pathol* 2003; 163: 1949–60.

51. Sell S. On the stem cell origin of cancer. *Am. J. Pathology* 2010; 176:2584–94.

52. Sell S. Stem cell origin of cancer and differentiation therapy. *Crit Rev Oncol Hematol* 2004; 51: 1–28.

53. Sell S. Leukemia: stem cells, maturation arrest and differentiation therapies. *Stem Cell Rev* 2005; 1: 197–205.

54. Muto A, Kizaki M, Yamato K, et al. 1,25 Dihydroxyvitamin D3 induces differentiation of a retinoic acid-resistent acute promyelocitic leukemia cell line (UF-1) associated with espression of p21 (WAF1/CIP1) and p 27 (K1P1). *Blood* 1999; 93: 2225–33.

55. Luo W, Yu WD, Ma Y, et al. Inhibition of protein kinase CK2 reduces Cyp24a1 expression and enhances 1,25-dihydroxyvitamin D (3) antitumor activity in human prostate cancer cells. *Cancer Res* 2013; 73: 2289–97.

56. Batie S, Lee JH, Jama RA, et al. Synthesis and biological evaluation of halogenated curcumin analogs as potential nuclear receptor selective agonists. *Bioorg Med Chem* 2013; 21: 693–702.

57. Sun SY, Lotan R. Retinoids and their receptors in cancer development and chemoprevention. *Crit. Rev Oncol Hematol* 2002, 41: 41–55.

58. Biava PM, Bonsignorio D, Hoxa M. Cell proliferation curves of different human tumor lines after in vitro treatment with Zebrafish embryonic extracts. *J Tumor Marker Oncol* 2001; 16: 195–202.

59. Biava PM, Carluccio A. Activation of anti-oncogene p53 produced by embryonic extracts in vitro tumor cells. *J Tumor Marker Oncol* 1977; 12: 9–15.

60. Biava PM, Bonsignorio D, Hoxa M, et al. Post-translational modification of the retinoblastoma protein (pRb) induced by in vitro administration of Zebrafish embryonic extracts on human kidney adenocarcinoma cell line. *J Tumor Marker Oncol* 2002; 17: 59–64.

61. Cucina A, Biava PM, D'Anselmi F, et al. Zebrafish embryo proteins induce apoptosis in human colon cancer cells (Caco2). *Apoptosis* 2006; 9: 1617–28.

62. D'Anselmi F, Cucina A, Biava PM, et al. Zebrafish stem cell differentiation stage factors suppress Bcl-xL release and enhance 5 Fu mediated apoptosis in colon cancer cells. *Curr Pharm Biotechnol* 2011; 12: 261–7.

63. Biava PM, Nicolini A, Ferrari P, Carpi A, Sell S. A systemic approach to cancer treatment: tumor cell reprogramming focused on endocrine-related cancers. *Current Med. Chem.* 2014, 21: 1072–81.

64. Livraghi T, Meloni F, Frosi A, Lazzaroni S, et al. Treatment with stem cell differentiation stage factors of intermediate-advanced hepatocellular carcinoma: an open randomized clinical trial. *Oncol Res* 2005; 15: 399–408.

65. Livraghi T, Ceriani R, Palmisano A, et al. Complete response in 5 out of 38 patients with advanced hepatocellular carcinoma treated with stem cell differentiation stage factors: case reports from a single centre. *Curr Pharm Biotechnol* 2011; 12: 254–60.

66. Allegrucci C, Rushton MD, Dixon JE, et al. Epigenetic reprogramming of breast cancer cells with oocyte extracts. *Mol Cancer* 2011; 10: 7.

67. Rachakatia RS, Troyer D. Wharton's jelly stromal cells as potential delivery vehicles for cancer therapeutics. *Future Oncol* 2009; 5: 1237–44.

68. Ganta C, Chiyo D, Ayuzawa R, et al. Rat umbical cord stem cells completely abolish rat mammary carcinomas with no evidence of metastasis or recurrence 100 days post-tumor cell inoculation. *Cancer Res* 2009; 69: 1815–20.

69. Xu T, Xu Y, Liao CP, Lau R, Goldkorn A. Reprogramming murine telomerase rapidly inhibits the growth of mouse cancer cells in vitro and in vivo. *Mol Cancer Ther* 2010; 9: 438–49.

70. Xu T, He K, Wang L, Goldkorn A. Prostate tumor cells with cancer progenitors properties have high telomerase activity and are rapidly killed by telomerase interference. *Prostate* 2011; 71: 1390–4000.

71. Xu Y, He K, Goldkorn A. Telomerase targeted therapy in cancer and cancer stem cells. *Clin Adv. Hematol Oncol* 2011; 9: 442–55.

72. Grzmil M, Voigt S, Thelen P, et al. Up-regulated expression of the MAT-8 gene in prostate cancer and its siRNA-mediated inhibition of expression induces a decrease in proliferation of human prostate carcinoma cells. *Int J Oncol* 2004; 24: 97–105.

73. Stolzenburg S, Rots MG, Beltran AS, et al. Targeted silencing of the oncogenic transcription factor SOX2 in breast cancer. *Nucleic Acids Res* 2012; 40: 6725–40.

74. Cubillos-Ruiz JR, Baird JR, Tesone AJ, et al. Reprogramming tumor-associated dendritic cells in vivo using miRNA mimetics triggers protective immunity against ovarian cancer. *Cancer Res* 2012; 72: 1683–93.

75. Quinn MC, Filali-Mouhim A, Provencher DM, Mes-Masson AM, Tonin PN. Reprogramming of the transcriptome in a novel chromosome 3 transfer tumor suppressor ovarian cancer cell line model affected molecular networks that are characteristic of ovarian cancer. *Mol Carcinog* 2009; 48: 648–61.

76. Biava PM, Bonsignorio D. Cancer and cell differentiation: a model to explain malignancy. *J Tumor Marker Oncol* 2002; 17: 47–54.

77. Shackeleton M, Quintana E, Fearon ER, Morrison SJ. Heterogeneity in cancer: cancer stem cells versus clonal evolution. *Cell* 2009; 138: 822–9.

78. Tang DG. Understanding cancer stem cell heterogeneity and plasticity. *Cell Res* 2012; 22: 457–72.

79. Visvader JE, Lindeman GJ. Cancer stem cells: current status and evolving complexities. *Cell Stem Cell* 2012; 10: 717–28.

80. Renan MJ. How many mutations are required for tumorigenesis? Implications from human cancer data. *Mol Carcinogenesis* 1993; 7: 139–46.

81. Han WC, Counter CM, Lundberg AS, et al. Creation of human tumor cells with defined genetic elements. *Nature* 1999; 400: 464–8.

82. Olumi AF, Grossfeld GD, Hayward SW, et al. Carcinoma associated fibroblasts direct tumor progression of initiated human prostatic epithelium. *Cancer Res* 1999; 59: 5002–11.

83. Hudson JD, Shoabi MA, Maestro R, et al. A proinflammatory cytokine inhibits p53 tumor suppressor activity. *J Exp Med* 1999; 190: 1375–82.

84. Hanahan D, Weinberg RA. The hallmarks of cancer. *Cell* 2000; 100: 57–70.

85. Biava PM, Monguzzi A, Bonsignorio D, et al. Xenopus Laevis embryo share antigens with Zebrafish embryos and with human malignant neoplasms. *J Tumor Marker Oncol* 2001; 16: 203–6.

86. Tannock IF. Cancer: Resistance through repopulation. *Nature* 2015; 517: 152–3.

87. Sato A, Sakurada K, Kumabe T, et al. Association of stem cell marker CD133 expression with dissemination of glioblastoma. *Neurosurg Rev* 2010; 33: 175–83.

88. Di Tommaso T, Mazzoleni S, Wang E, et al. Immunobiological characterization of cancer stem cells isolated from glioblastoma patients. *Cli. Cancer Res* 2010; 16: 800–13.

89. Ji J, Black KL, Yu JS. Glioma stem cell research for the development of immunotherapy. *Neurosurg Clin N Am* 2010: 21: 159–66.

90. Chen J, Chen ZL. Technology update for the sorting and identification of breast cancer stem cells. *Chin J Cancer* 2010; 29: 265–9.

91. Park SY, Lee HE, Li H, et al. Heterogeneity for stem cell-related markers according to tumor subtype and histologic stage in breast cancer. *Cancer Res* 2010; 16: 876–87.

92. Lawson JC, Blatch GL, Edkins AL. Cancer stem cells in breast cancer and metastasis. *Cancer Res Treat* 2009; 8: 241–54.

93. Luo J, Yin X, Ma T, Lu J. Stem cells in normal mammary gland and breast cancer. *Am J Med Sci* 2010; 339: 366–70.

94. Spiro SG, Tanner NT, Silvestri GA, et al. Lung cancer: progress in diagnosis staging and therapy. *Respirology* 2010; 15: 44–50.

95. Gorelik E, Lokshin A, Levina L. Lung cancer stem cells as target for therapy. *Anticancer Agents Med Chem* 2010; 10: 164–71.

96. Sullivan JP, Minna JD, Shay JW. Evidence for self-renewing lung cancer stem cells and their implications in tumor initiation, progression and targeted therapy. *Cancer Metastasis Rev* 2010; 29: 61–72.

97. Westhoff B, Colaluca IN, D'Ario G, et al. Alteration of the Notch pathway in lung cancer. *Proc Natl Acad Sci USA* 2010; 87: 457–66.

98. Lawson DA, Zong Y, Memarzadeh S, et al. Basal epithelial stem cells are efficient targets for prostate cancer initiation. *Proc Natl Acad Sci USA* 2010; 107: 2610–15.

99. Lang SH, Anderson E, Fordham R, Collin AT. Modeling the prostate stem cell niche: an evaluation of stem cell survival and expansion in vitro. *Stem Cell Rev* 2010; 19: 537–46.

100. Joung JY, Cho KS, Kim JE, et al. Prostate stem cell antigen mRNA in peripheral blood as a potential predictor of biochemical recurrence of metastatic prostate cancer. *J Surg Oncol* 2010; 101: 145–8.

101. Liu T, Cheng W, Lai D, Huang Y, Guo L. Characterization of primary ovarian cancer cells in different culture systems. *Oncol Rep* 2010; 23: 1277–84.

102. Fong MY, Kakar SS. The role of cancer stem cells and the side population in epithelial ovarian cancer. *Histol. Histopatol* 2010; 25: 113–20.

103. Murphy SK. Targeting ovarian cancer initiating cells. *Anticancer Agents Med Chem* 2010; 10: 157–63.

104. Pen S, Maihle NJ, Huang Y. Pluripotency factors Lin 28 and Oct 4 identify a sub-population of stem cell-like cells in ovarian cancer. *Oncogene* 2010; 29: 2153–59.

105. Zou GM. Liver cancer stem cells as an important target in liver cancer therapies. *Anticancer Agents Med Chem* 2010; 10: 172–175.

106. Lee TK, Castilho A, Ma S, Ng IO. Liver cancer stem cells: implication for new therapeutic target. *Liver Int* 2009; 29: 955–65.

107. Marquardt JU, Thorgeirsson SS. Stem Cells in hepatocarcinogenesis: evidence from genomic data. *Semin Liver Dis* 2010; 30: 26–34.

108. Kung JW, Currie IS, Forbes SJ, Ross JA. Liver development, regeneration, and carcinogenesis. *J Biomed Biotechnol* 2010; 30: 26–34.

109. Gai H, Nguyen DM, Moon YJ, et al. Generation of murine hepatic lineage cells from induced pluripotent stem cells. *Differentiation* 2010; 79: 171–81.

110. Nishii T, Yashiro M, Shinto O, et al. Cancer stem cell-like SP cells have a high adhesion ability to the peritoneum in gastric carcinoma. *Cancer Sci* 2009; 100: 1397–402.

111. Chen Z, Xu WR, Quian H, et al. Oct4 a novel marker for human gastric cancer. *J Surg Oncol* 2009; 34: 1201–7.

112. Kang DH, Han ME, Song MH, et al. The role of hedgehog signaling during gastric regeneration. *J Gastroenterol* 2009; 44: 372–9.

113. Correia M, Machado JC, Ristimaki A. Basic aspects of gastric cancer. *Helicobacter* 2009; 14: 36–40.

114. Takaishi S, Okumura T, Tu S, et al. Identification of gastric cancer stem cells using the surface marker CD44. *Stem Cells* 2009; 59: 106–20.

115. Nishii T, Yashiro M, Shinto O, et al. Cancer stem cell-like SP cells have a high adhesion ability to the peritoneum in gastric carcinoma. *Cancer Sci* 2009; 100: 1397–402.

116. Yeung TM, Ghandhi SC, Wilding JL, Muschel R, Bodmer WF. Cancer stem cells from colorectal cancer derived cell lines. *Proc Natl Acad Sci USA* 2010; 107: 3722–7.

117. Gulino A, Ferretti E, De Smaele E. Hedgehog signaling in colon cancer and stem cells. *EMBO Mol Med* 2009; 1: 300–2.

118. Thenappen A, Li Y, Shetty K, et al. New therapeutic targeting colon cancer stem cells. *Curr Colorectal Cancer Rep* 2009; 5: 209.

119. Rasheed ZA, Yang J, Wang Q, et al. Prognostic significance of tumorigenic cells with mesenchymal features in pancreatic adenocarcinoma. *J Natl Cancer Inst* 2010; 102: 340–51.

120. Puri S, Hebrok M. Cellular plasticity within pancreas-lessons learned from development. *Dev Cell* 2010; 18: 342–56.

121. Quante M, Wang TC. Stem cells in gastroenterology and hepatology. *Nat Rev Gastroenterol Hepatol* 2009; 6: 724–37.

122. Ailles L, Prince M. Cancer stem cells in head and neck squamous cell carcinoma. *Methods Mol Biol* 2009; 568: 175–93.

123. Zhang P, Zhang Y, Mao L, Zhang Z, Chen W. Side population in oral squamous cell carcinoma possesses tumor stem cell phenotype. *Cancer Lett* 2009; 277: 227–34.

124. Brunner M, Thurnher D, Heiduschka G, et al. Elevated levels of circulating endothelial progenitor cells in head and neck cancer patients. *J Surg Oncol* 2008; 98: 545–50.

125. Zhang Q, Shi S, Yen Y, et al. A subpopulation of CD133(+) cancer stem-like cells characterized in human oral squamous cell carcinoma confer resistance to chemotherapy. *Cancer Lett* 2010; 289: 151–60.

126. Strizzi L, Postovit LM, Margaryan NV, et al. Nodal as biomarker for melanoma progression and a new therapeutic target for clinical intervention. *Expert Rev Dermatol* 2009; 4: 67–78.

127. Hanahan D, Weinberg RA. Hallmarks of cancer: the next generation. *Cell* 2011; 144: 646–74.

128. Biava PM, Nicolini A, Ferrari P, Carpi A, Sell S. Systemic approach to cancer treatment: tumor cell reprogramming focused on endocrine-related cancers. *Current Med Chem* 2014; 21: 1072–81.

ABSTRACTS OF SELECTED STUDIES

Stem Cell Differentiation Stage Factors and Their Role in Triggering Symmetry Breaking Processes during Cancer Development: A Quantum Field Theory Model for Reprogramming Cancer Cells to Healthy Phenotypes

Current Medicinal Chemistry, 2017 Sept 20

P. M. Biava, F. Burigana, R. Germano, P. Kurian,
C. Verzegnassi, G. Vitiello

This study interprets results obtained using stem cell differentiation stage factors for reprogramming tumor cells in light of quantum field theory. It examines the effects of reprogramming tumor cells not only in light of the effects on biochemical mechanisms studied in the laboratory, but also in modulating electrochemical phenomena and electrodynamic behavior regarding the molecules of a network of differentiation factors and interstitial water. The study describes how changes in the genetic and epigenetic code are transmitted and amplified in the microenvironment of tumor cell populations, and how changes in the information field of the microenvironment can be used to reprogram tumor cells to healthy, non-proliferative states. Recent investigations have shown that proteins are capable of finding their cognate partners ten and even a hundred times faster than predicted by the Brownian diffusion rates, suggesting that electromagnetic effects can critically affect the time needed for two biomolecular partners to encounter each other.

A long history of research has pursued the use of embryonic factors isolated during cell differentiation processes for the express purpose of transforming cancer cells back to healthy phenotypes. Recent results have clarified that the substances present at different stages of cell differentiation—which we call stem cell differentiation stage factors (SCDSFs)—are proteins with low molecular weight and nucleic acids that regulate genomic expression. The present review summarizes how these substances, taken at different stages of cellular maturation, are able to retard proliferation of many human tumor cell lines and thereby reprogram cancer cells to healthy phenotypes. The model presented here is a quantum field theory (QFT) model in which SCDSFs are able to trigger symmetry breaking processes during cancer development.

These symmetry breaking processes, which lie at the root of many phenomena in elementary particle and condensed-matter physics, govern the phase transitions of totipotent cells to higher degrees of diversity and order, resulting in cell differentiation. In cancers, which share many genomic and metabolic similarities with embryonic stem cells, stimulated re-differentiation often signifies the phenotypic reversion back to health and non-proliferation. In addition to acting on key components of the cellular cycle, SCDSFs are able to reprogram cancer cells by delicately influencing the cancer microenvironment, modulating the electrochemistry and thus the collective electrodynamic behaviors between dipole networks in biomacromolecules and the interstitial water field. Coherent effects in biological water, which are derived from a dissipative QFT framework, may offer new diagnostic and therapeutic targets at a systemic level, before tumor instantiation occurs in specific tissues or organs. Thus, by including the environment as an essential component of our model, we may push the prevailing paradigm of mutation-driven oncogenesis toward a closer description of reality.

The Role of Neuroendocrine Cells in Prostate Cancer: A Comprehensive Review of Current Literature and Subsequent Rationale to Broaden and Integrate Current Treatment Modalities

---

Current Medicinal Chemistry, 2014, Volume 21, Number 9: 1082–92.

F. Lugnani, G. Simone, P. M. Biava, R. J. Ablin

Neuroendocrine prostate carcinoma (NE-PCa) is a heterogeneous disease. Due to a high prevalence of NE (neuroendocrine) differentiation in patients who receive prolonged androgen deprivation treatment, the real incidence of NE-PCa remains unknown. Similarly, the biological steps from prostate carcinoma (PCa) toward NE differentiation are far less than definitive and, consequently, there is a lack of evidence to support any of the treatments as the "gold standard."

Materials and Methods

A systematic literature search was conducted using the PubMed, Scopus, and Embase databases to identify original articles and review articles regarding NE-PCa. Keywords were "prostate cancer" and "neuroendocrine." Articles published between 1995 and 2013 were reviewed and selected with the consensus of all of the authors.

Results

Fifty-one articles were selected by the authors for the purpose of this review. The principle findings were reported into some subsections: Epidemiology, Biological steps of NE differentiation (with some principle articles on animal and in vitro, since there is very little in the literature on human studies); for the treatment options, we had to expand the search on PubMed to a larger timeframe and selection since very little was specifically found in the first criteria: surgery, radiotherapy, ablative techniques, immunomodulation, and epigenetic therapy were then reviewed. A multidisciplinary approach, advocated by many authors, although promising, has failed to demonstrate increased survival rates. Limitations of this review include the lack of a clear definition of NE-PCa and, consequently, the lack of strong evidence provided by a large series with long-term follow-up.

Conclusions

Supported by this extensive review, we propose it is worthwhile to investigate a new multimodal therapeutic approach to address advanced NE-PCa starting from a debunking (with radical intent) of the disease plus epigenetic therapy with stem cell differentiation stage factors

(SCDSFs). In addition, immunotherapy can be used to treat the cancer presenting phenotype in association with chemomodulation plus ablative therapies, in case of advanced or recurrent diseases. SCDSFs may be utilized to regulate cancer stem cells, and possible new phenotypes could also be associated with ablative therapies. Hormonal deprivation, radiotherapy, chemotherapy, ex vivo vaccines and targeted therapies could also be used and reserved in case of failure.

A Systemic Approach to Cancer Treatment: Tumor Cell Reprogramming Focused on Endocrine-Related Cancers

Current Medicinal Chemistry, 2014, Volume 21, Number 9: 1072–81.

P. M. Biava, A. Nicolini, P. Ferrari, A. Carpi, S. Sell

The term "cancer cell reprogramming" is used to define any kind of intervention aimed at transforming cancer cells into terminally differentiated cells. Using this approach, new technologies have been applied with different methods for a more systemic approach to cancer treatment. This review reports on advances of these technologies, including our personal contributions, mainly carried out on endocrine-related cancers. Some of the interventions, aimed at reverting cancer cells into a normal phenotype, are based on the evidence that tumor development is suppressed by the embryonic microenvironment. On the basis of this rationale, experiments have been conducted using stem cell differentiation stage factors (SCDSFs) taken at different stages of development of Zebrafish embryos, oocyte extracts, or naive human umbilical cord matrix derived stem cells (UMDSCs). SCDSFs induce significant growth inhibition on different tumor cell lines in vitro, likely because of increases in cell cycle regulatory molecules, such as p53 and pRb.

Treatment with these factors activates apoptosis and differentiation related to caspase-3. This is achieved via p73 apoptotic-dependent pathway activation with a concurrent normalization of the E-cadherin and beta-catenin ratio. Extracts from prophase amphibian oocytes could reprogram relevant epigenetic alterations in MCF-7 and HCC1954 breast cancer cell lines, while un-engineered (naive) human UMDSCs attenuated growth of MDA-231 human breast carcinoma cells. A product prepared for human treatments, containing SCDSFs at very low doses, yielded favorable results in breast cancer and in intermediate-advanced hepatocellular carcinoma. Other reprogramming interventions used in the models of breast, prostate, and ovarian cancer cell lines are described. Finally, current and future perspectives of this novel technology are discussed, and a new hallmark of cancer is suggested: the loss of differentiation of cancer cells.

The Zebrafish Embryo Derivative Affects Cell Viability of Epidermal Cells: A Possible Role in the Treatment of Psoriasis

Giornale Italiano di Dermatologia e Venereologia, 2013 October, Volume 148, Number 5: 479–83.

G. D. Norata, P. M. Biava, F. Di Pierro

In patients affected by psoriasis, use of a topical formula containing a derivative of Zebrafish embryos was associated with reduced skin inflammation and dermal turnover, as well as a generally better outcome. In an attempt to understand the molecular mechanisms lying beyond these findings, we investigated the anti-proliferative effects of the Zebrafish embryo derivative by addressing the mitochondrial function (MTT assay) and cell nuclei distribution (Hoestch staining). In cell cultures stimulated with fetal calf serum (FCS) or epidermal growth factor (EGF), the Zebrafish derivative significantly inhibited cell proliferation induced by either approach, although the effect was stronger in cells stimulated with FCS. These results suggest that the Zebrafish embryo derivative may dampen increased cell proliferation; this obser-

vation may be relevant to cutaneous pathologies related to altered proliferative mechanisms, including psoriasis.

Cancer Cell Reprogramming:
Stem Cell Differentiation Stage Factors
and an Agent-Based Model to Optimize Cancer Treatment

Current Pharmaceutical Biotechnology, 2011,
Volume 12, Number 2: 231–242.

P. M. Biava, M. Basevi, L. Biggiero, A. Borgonovo,
E. Borgonovo, F. Burigana

Recent tumor research has led scientists to recognize the central role played by cancer stem cells in sustaining malignancy and
chemoresistance. A model of cancer presented by one of us describes
the mechanisms that give rise to the different kinds of cancer stem-
like cells and the role of these cells in cancer diseases. The model
implies a shift in the conceptualization of the disease from reductionism to complexity theory. By exploiting the link between the agent-
based simulation technique and the theory of complexity, the medical
view is here translated into a corresponding computational model.
Two main categories of agents characterize the model: 1) cancer stem-
like cells and 2) stem cell differentiation stage factors. Cancer cells
agents are then distinguished based on the differentiation stage associated with the malignancy. Differentiation factors interact with cancer
cells and then, with varying degrees of fitness, induce differentiation
or cause apoptosis. The model inputs are then fitted to experimental data and numerical simulations carried out. By performing virtual
experiments on the model's choice variables, a decision-maker (physician) can obtain insights on the progression of the disease and on
the effects of a choice of administration frequency and or dose. The
model also paves the way to future research, whose perspectives are
discussed.

Zebrafish Stem Cell Differentiation Stage Factors Suppress Bcl-Xl, Release and Enhance 5-Fu-Mediated Apoptosis in Colon Cancer Cells

Current Pharmaceutical Biotechnology, 2011, Volume 12, Number 2: 261–267

F. D'Anselmi, A. Cucina, P. M. Biava, S. Proietti, P. Coluccia, L. Frati, M. Bizzarri

Stem cell differentiation stage factors (SCDSF), taken from Zebrafish embryos during the stage in which totipotent stem cells are differentiating into pluripotent stem cells, have been shown to inhibit proliferation and induce apoptosis in colon tumors. In order to ascertain if these embryonic factors could synergistically/additively interact with 5-Fluorouracil (5-Fu), whole cell-count, flow-cytometry analysis, and apoptotic parameters were recorded in human colon cancer cells (Caco2) treated with Zebrafish stem cell differentiation stage factors (SCDSF 3 µg/ml) in association or not with 5-Fu in the sub-pharmacological therapeutic range (0.01 mg/ml). Cell proliferation was significantly reduced by SCDSF, while SCDSF+5-Fu leads to an almost complete growth-inhibition. SCDSF produces a significant apoptotic effect, while the association with 5-FU leads to an enhanced additive apoptotic rate at both 24 and 72 hrs. SCDSF alone and in association with 5-Fu triggers both the extrinsic and the intrinsic apoptotic pathways, activating caspase-8, -3 and -7. SCDSF and 5-Fu alone exerted opposite effects on Bax and Bcl-xL proteins; meanwhile, SCDSF+5-Fu induced an almost complete suppression of Bcl-xL release and a dramatic increase in the Bax/Bcl-xL ratio. These data suggest that Zebrafish embryo factors could improve chemotherapy efficacy by reducing anti-apoptotic proteins involved in drug-resistance processes.

Embryonic Morphogenetic Fields Induce Phenotypic Reversion in Cancer Cells

Current Pharmaceutical Biotechnology, 2011,
Volume 12, Number 2: 243–253.

M. Bizzarri, A. Cucina, P. M. Biava, S. Proietti, et al.

Cancer cells introduced into developing embryos can be committed to a complete reversion of their malignant phenotype. It is unlikely that such effects could be ascribed to only a few molecular components interacting according to a simple linear-dynamics model, and they claim against the somatic mutation theory of cancer. Some 50 years ago, Needham and Waddington speculated that cancer represents an escape from a morphogenetic field like those that guide embryonic development. Indeed, disruption of the morphogenetic field of a tissue can promote the onset as well as the progression of cancer. On the other hand, placing tumor cells into a "normal" morphogenetic field—like that of an embryonic tissue—one can reverse malignant phenotype, "reprogramming" tumor into normal cells. According to the theoretical framework provided by the thermodynamics of dissipative systems, morphogenetic fields could be considered as distinct attractors, to which cell behaviors are converging. Cancer-attractors are likely positioned somewhat close to embryonic-attractors. Indeed, tumors share several morphological and ultra-structural features with embryonic cells. The recovering of an "embryonic-like" cell shape might enable the gene regulatory network to reactivate embryonic programs, and consequently to express antigenic and biochemical embryonic characters. This condition confers to cancer an unusual sensitivity to embryonic regulatory cues. Thus, it is not surprising that cancer cells exposed to specific embryonic morphogenetic fields undergo significant modifications, eventually leading to a complete phenotypic reversion.

Cancer, Cell Death, and Differentiation:
The Role of Epigenetic Code in Tumor Growth Control

A Nature Conference:

Cancer Therapeutics: The Road Ahead

October 8–10, 2007, Palazzo dei Congressi di Capri (Italy)

P. M. Biava of Foundation for Research into the Biological Therapies of Cancer, IRCCS Multimedica (Milano)

A. Frosi of Hepatology-Gastroenterology Unit, Sesto S. G. Hospital (Milano)

M. Bizzarri and L. Frati of Department of Experimental Medicine and Pathology, Università La Sapienza (Roma)

Experiments on different human tumor cell lines (glioblastoma multiforme, melanoma, breast carcinoma, kidney adenocarcinoma, colon adenocarcinoma, acute lymphoblastic leukemia) treated with stem cell differentiation stage factors taken from Zebrafish embyos during the stage of cell differentiation, in which totipotent stem cells differentiate into pluripotent stem cells, demonstrated a significant slowdown in tumor proliferation rate. The same results were obtained when tumor cells were treated with factors present in other different cell differentiation stages of Zebrafish embryos, like 5 somites and 20 somites stages, whereas no slowing effect was observed when tumor cells were treated with the factors taken from a merely multiplicative stage, like morula. In addition we observed a significant decrease in Lewis Lung Carcinoma injected in C57BL/6 mice treated with differentiation factors. Thus cell differentiation could be viewed as a key process in controlling the behavior of tumor cells. Our studies carried out in order to find out which cell regulation pathways are involved in the embryo in this mechanism of tumor growth demonstrated that key role cell cycle regulator molecules, such as p53 and pRb are modified by transcriptional and post-translational processes. Research on apoptosis and differentiation revealed that treatment with stem cell differentiation stage factors induces caspase 3 activation, mainly by increasing the releases of E2F-1, leading to c-Myc overexpression and activation of a p73 apoptotic-dependent pathway. Moreover, a concurrent significant normalization effect on the ratio of e-cadherin/beta catenin expression with increase in e-cadherin levels was observed (data not yet published). Finally, a product prepared for human therapy containing stem cell differentiation stage factors demonstrated 19.8% regression, 16% stable diseases, and a significant difference in survival between the group of patients who responded to treatment versus the group with progression disease (p<0.001) in an open randomized clinical trial on 179 consecutive patients with intermediate-advanced hepatocellular carcinoma. On the basis of these studies, a new vision of cancer related to a complexity model was proposed, confirming the importance of epigenetic modulation by factors present during precise stages of cell differentiation in controlling tumor growth.

Zebrafish Embryo Proteins Induce Apoptosis in Human Colon Cancer Cells (Caco2)

Apoptosis, 2006 September, Volume 11, Number 9: 1617–28.

A. Cucina, P. M. Biava, F. D'Anselmi, P. Coluccia, F. Conti, R. di Clemente, A. Miccheli, L. Frati, A. Gulino, M. Bizzarri

Previous studies have shown that proteins extracted from Zebrafish embryo share some cytostatic characteristics in cancer cells. Our study was conducted to ascertain the biological properties of this protein network. Cancer cell growth and apoptosis were studied in Caco2 cells treated with embryonic extracts. Cell proliferation was significantly inhibited in a dose-dependent manner. Cell-cycle analysis in treated cells revealed a marked accumulation in the G(2)/M phase preceding induction of apoptosis. Embryo proteins induced a significant reduction in FLIP levels and increased caspase-3 and caspase-8 activity as well as the apoptotic rate. Increased phosphorylated pRb values were obtained in treated Caco2 cells: the modified balance in pRb phosphorylation was associated with an increase in E2F1 values and c-Myc over-expression. Our data support previous reports of an apoptotic enhancing effect displayed by embryo extracts, mainly through the pRb/E2F1 apoptotic pathway, which thus suggests that Zebrafish embryo proteins have complex anti-cancer properties.

Treatment with Stem Cell Differentiation Stage Factors of Intermediate-Advanced Hepatocellular Carcinoma: An Open Randomized Clinical Trial

Oncology Research, 2005, Volume 15, Number 7-8: 399–408

T. Livraghi, F. Meloni, A. Frosi, S. Lazzaroni, M. Bizzarri,
L. Frati, P. M. Biava

Corresponding Author: P. M. Biava

There is no standard treatment for patients with advanced hepato-cellular carcinoma (HCC). We developed a product containing stem cells differentiation stage factors (SCDSF) that inhibits tumor growth in vivo and in vitro. The aim of this open randomized study was to assess its efficacy in patients with HCC not suitable for resection, transplantation, ablation therapy, or arterial chemoembolization. A total of 179 consecutive patients were enrolled. We randomly assigned the patients to receive either SCDSF or only conservative treatment. Primary end points were tumor response and survival. Secondary end points were performance status and patient tolerance. Randomization was stopped at the second interim analysis (6 months) of the first 32 patients recruited when the inspection detected a significant difference in favor of treatment (p = 0.037). The responses to the therapy obtained in 154 additional patients confirmed previous results. Evaluation of survival showed a significant difference between the group of patients who responded to treatment versus the group with progression of disease (p<0.001). Of the 23 treated patients with a performance status (PS) of 1, 19 changed to 0. The study indicated the efficacy of SCDSF treatment of the patients with intermediate-advanced HCC.

About the Authors

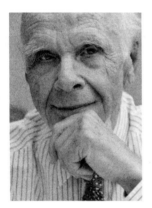

Ervin Laszlo, Ph.D., is a philosopher and systems scientist. Twice nominated for the Nobel Peace Prize, he has published more than 75 books and over 400 articles and research papers. The subject of the one-hour PBS special *The Life of a Modern-Day Genius,* Laszlo is the founder and president of the international think tank the Club of Budapest and of the prestigious Laszlo Institute of New Paradigm Research. The winner of the 2017 Luxembourg Peace Prize, he lives in Tuscany.

Laszlo's Books on the New Paradigm

The Connectivity Hypothesis
Foundations of an Integral Science of Quantum, Cosmos, Life, and Consciousness
Albany: State University of New York Press, 2003

Science and the Akashic Field
An Integral Theory of Everything
Rochester, VT: Inner Traditions International, 2004

Science and the Reenchantment of the Cosmos
The Rise of the Integral Vision of Reality
Rochester, VT: Inner Traditions International, 2008

Quantum Shift in the Global Brain
How the New Scientific Reality Can Change Us and Our World
Rochester, VT: Inner Traditions International, 2008

The Akashic Experience
Science and the Cosmic Memory Field
Rochester, VT: Inner Traditions International, 2009

The Dawn of the Akashic Age
New Consciousness, Quantum Resonance, and the Future of the World
with Kingsley Dennis
Rochester, VT: Inner Traditions International, 2013

Il Senso Ritrovato
with Pier Mario Biava
Milan: Springer (in Italian), 2013

The Self-Actualizing Cosmos
The Akasha Revolution in Science and Human Consciousness
Rochester, VT: Inner Traditions International, 2014

The Immortal Mind
Science and the Continuity of Consciousness Beyond the Brain
with Anthony Peake
Rochester, VT: Inner Traditions International, 2014

What Is Consciousness
Three Sages Lift the Veil
with Larry Dossey and Jean Houston
New York: Select Books, 2016

What Is Reality?
The New Map of Cosmos and Consciousness
New York: Select Books, 2016

The Intelligence of the Cosmos
Why Are We Here—New Answers from the Frontiers of Science
Rochester, VT: Inner Traditions, 2017

The Handbook of New Paradigm Research
Cardiff, CA: Waterside Press, 2018

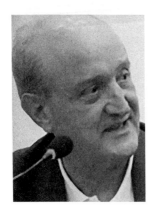

Pier Mario Biava, M.D., has been studying the relationship between cancer and cell differentiation for more than three decades. The author of over 100 scientific publications and eight books, he works at the Institute of Research and Treatment in Milan.

Biava's Books on the New Discovery

L'aggressione Nascosta. Limiti Sanitari Di Esposizione Ai Rischi
Milan: Feltrinelli, 1981

Complessità E Biologia
with M Gellman et al.
Milan: Mondadori, 2002

Il Cancro E La Ricerca Del Senso Perduto
New York: Springer, 2008

Cancer and the Search for Lost Meaning
Berkeley: North Atlantic Books, 2009

Il Senso Ritrovato
with Ervin Laszlo
New York: Springer, 2012

Dal Segno Al Simbolo. Il Manifesto Del Nuovo Paradigma In Medicina
with Ervin Laszlo and D. Frigoli
Bologna: Persiani, 2014

Parlare Al Cancro. La Ricerca Del Dialogo Per Riprogrammare Le Cellule
with Nader Butto et al.
Cervia, Italy: Eifis, 2017

Happygenetica
with R. Romagnoli
Cervia, Italy: Eifis, 2017

Index

Page numbers in *italics* indicate illustrations

BOOKS OF RELATED INTEREST

Science and the Akashic Field
An Integral Theory of Everything
by Ervin Laszlo

The Intelligence of the Cosmos
Why Are We Here? New Answers from the Frontiers of Science
by Ervin Laszlo
Foreword by Jane Goodall

The Cosmic Hologram
In-formation at the Center of Creation
by Jude Currivan, Ph.D.
Foreword by Ervin Laszlo

The Miracle of Regenerative Medicine
How to Naturally Reverse the Aging Process
by Elisa Lottor, Ph.D., HMD
Foreword by Judi Goldstone, M.D.

Quantum DNA Healing
Consciousness Techniques for Altering Your Genetic Destiny
by Althea S. Hawk

Structural Integration and Energy Medicine
A Handbook of Advanced Bodywork
by Jean Louise Green
Foreword by James L. Oschman, Ph.D.

The Science of Planetary Signatures in Medicine
Restoring the Cosmic Foundations of Healing
by Jennifer T. Gehl, MHS
With Marc S. Micozzi, M.D., Ph.D.

Vibrational Medicine
The #1 Handbook of Subtle-Energy Therapies
by Richard Gerber, M.D.

INNER TRADITIONS • BEAR & COMPANY
P.O. Box 388
Rochester, VT 05767
1-800-246-8648
www.InnerTraditions.com

Or contact your local bookseller